Contents

About the authors

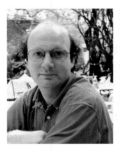

Dr M.C. Walker, PhD, MRCP is a Senior Lecturer in Neurology at the Institute of Neurology, UCL and also Consultant at the National Hospital for Neurology and Neurosurgery, London.

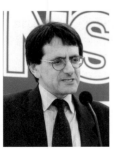

Professor Simon Shorvon, MD, FCRP is Professor of Clinical Neurology at the Institute of Neurology, UCL and Consultant Neurologist at the National Hospital for Neurology and Neurosurgery, London.

Introduction

How long has epilepsy been known?

What do the following people have in common: Julius Caesar, the apostle St Paul, Dostoyevski, van Gogh, the prophet Mohammed, Joan of Arc, Buddha, Edward Lear, Gustav Flaubert and Alexander the Great? The answer is that they probably all had epilepsy.

Why do we try to hide it?

Today there are people from all walks of life who have epilepsy. It is therefore somewhat surprising that prejudices or stigmatisation results in many people hiding their epilepsy from friends, employers and sometimes even members of their own family.

Unpredictable and frightening

Epilepsy has undoubtedly achieved its unenviable position in people's minds perhaps, largely, because of its unpredictable, dramatic and sometimes frightening effects. Although there are many different types of seizures, as explained later, it is the convulsion – falling to the ground, frothing at the mouth, flailing of the limbs – that comes to most people's minds when the word epilepsy is mentioned.

Historical beliefs

It is this dramatic event that has always fuelled people's imaginations; epileptic seizures are mentioned in the earliest Babylonian and Hebrew tracts. In Ancient Greece, at a time obsessed with gods and spirits, Hippocrates was one of the first to try to dispel the mysticism of epileptic seizures. He firmly believed that epilepsy originated in the brain and even went as far as condemning those charlatans who proposed that epilepsy was caused by demonic possession.

Yet, for the next 2,000 years, it was this theory of demonic possession that led to people with epilepsy being shunned, locked away, and subjected to painful and humiliating ordeals in the name of a cure.

Historical treatments

In the account of the death of Charles II, there is a description of the treatment of his seizure; this included bleeding him, giving him substances that made him sick and repeated enemas, shaving his head, blistering his skin and then finally forcing an unpleasant concoction down the dying king's throat.

Even as recently as the nineteenth century, circumcision and castration were proposed as cures of epilepsy. It was not until the end of the nineteenth century that the first effective drug, potassium bromide, was introduced, and from that time drug treatment has allowed most people with epilepsy to lead normal, seizure-free lives.

Modern attitudes

There is still, to a certain extent, a stigma attached to what is a common condition (almost every one of us knows someone who has epilepsy, although we may not realise that he or she has the condition). In modern society, stigma usually relates to a fear of the unknown, a fear of 'madness', the apparent loss of control, the anxiety to an onlooker that seizures are a prelude to death, or the associated inconvenience and embarrassment.

How common is epilepsy?

Epilepsy is very common. Each year in the United Kingdom about 25,000 people develop epilepsy; most are either children or elderly people (epilepsy infrequently starts between the ages of 20 and 50).

There is about a 1 in 30 chance of developing epilepsy during a lifetime. However, only 1 in 200 people has active epilepsy (350,000 people in the UK). This implies that most people with epilepsy get better, and indeed this is the case; in about 6 of every 10 people the condition resolves.

How many people have epilepsy?

Epilepsy is very common. There is about a 1 in 30 chance of developing it at some time. Of 50 million people, the approximate population of the UK:

- 1,000,000–2,500,000 will develop epilepsy in their lifetime
- 250,000–500,000 will have active epilepsy
- 10,000–35,000 will develop epilepsy each year

Epilepsy affects males and females almost equally, although certain types of epilepsy are more common in one or other sex. It affects all classes and all races.

Thus, epilepsy is common and treatment is frequently successful, This is an important message for all those who develop it.

KEY POINTS

- There are many types of epilepsy and seizures
- Epilepsy usually begins in childhood or old age
- Epilepsy is common, but usually resolves

What are seizures and epilepsy?

A short definition

Epilepsy is usually defined as a condition in which the person is liable to have recurrent epileptic seizures. Epileptic seizures (or fits as they are sometimes known) can take a variety of forms, depending on where in the brain they arise.

How is the brain involved?
Brain organisation

The brain is involved in forming emotions, thoughts and memories, in controlling movement, and in appreciating sensations, sounds, smells, tastes and sight. It is divided into two halves joined in the middle: the right half controls motor and sensory function of the left-hand side of the body and the left half controls the right-hand side.

For most of us, the left half is also 'dominant' – in other words, it controls how we form and understand language. Each half (or hemisphere) is further divided into four lobes as shown in the diagram.

The structure of the brain

The brain has two hemispheres: the left and the right. Each hemisphere is composed of four lobes. Each of the four lobes of each cerebral hemisphere has its own particular physical and mental functions. These can be impaired by brain damage.

SIDE VIEW

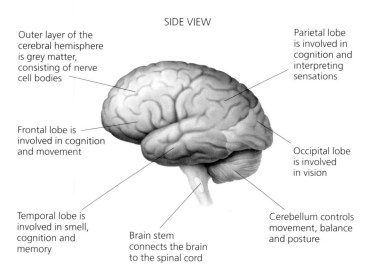

Outer layer of the cerebral hemisphere is grey matter, consisting of nerve cell bodies

Parietal lobe is involved in cognition and interpreting sensations

Frontal lobe is involved in cognition and movement

Occipital lobe is involved in vision

Temporal lobe is involved in smell, cognition and memory

Brain stem connects the brain to the spinal cord

Cerebellum controls movement, balance and posture

TOP VIEW

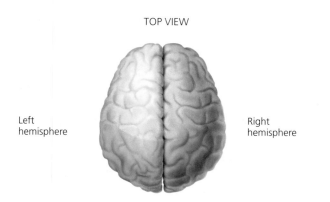

Left hemisphere

Right hemisphere

The structure of the brain

The brain has two hemispheres: the left and right. Each hemisphere is composed of four lobes. Each of the four lobes of each cerebral hemisphere has its own particular physical and mental functions. These can be impaired by brain damage or overactivated by brain stimulation.

What happens if part of the brain is damaged?

Damage to one part of the brain will take away its function. For example, damage to the left occipital lobe will result in the person being unable to see anything on the right; damage to the right frontal lobe may cause a person to be paralysed down the left-hand side.

What happens if the brain is activated?

Conversely, activation, such as that which occurs in an epileptic seizure, results in an exaggeration of normal function. Thus, for instance, an epileptic seizure occurring in the left occipital lobe will result in abnormal visual perceptions (coloured lights, visions, etc.), and seizure occurring in the right frontal lobe will result in abnormal movements of the left side of the body.

What happens to the brain in a seizure?

A seizure can be likened to an electrical storm. This storm can be confined to one part of the brain, spread to other parts of the brain or involve the whole brain at once. Those that start in one part of the brain are known as 'partial seizures' and those that start in both halves at once are known as 'generalised seizures'. What is experienced depends on where in the brain the seizure starts, and how far and how quickly it spreads.

The next section defines the different types of seizure in some detail.

Types of seizures

Almost all seizures are sudden, short-lived and self-limiting. Most occur spontaneously without warning and, as explained above, the form of the seizure depends on the part of the brain involved. The classification is presented in the box.

Partial seizures

Simple partial seizures

These are seizures confined to one small part of the brain, during which there is no loss of consciousness. They are often divided into temporal lobe, frontal lobe,

---

Classification of seizures

There are many types of seizure in epilepsy. All come on suddenly and don't last long. The form a seizure takes depends on which parts of the brain are involved.

Partial seizures	A	Simple partial seizures
	B	Complex partial seizures
	C	Secondary generalised seizures
Generalised seizures	A	Absence seizures (petit mal)
	B	Myoclonic seizures
	C	Clonic seizures
	D	Tonic seizures
	E	Tonic–clonic seizures (grand mal)
	F	Atonic seizures

parietal lobe and occipital lobe seizures, depending on where the seizure starts:

- In temporal lobe seizures, the patient may experience a feeling of intense fear, vivid memory flash-backs, intense déjà vu (a feeling of having been in an identical situation before), a rising sensation and unpleasant intense smells or tastes. We can all experience some of these from time to time and of course they are not usually seizures; for example, déjà vu is a common and normal experience.

  The main difference is that, with epilepsy, these things happen regularly, without reason, are short-lived and occur with an intensity that is rare in everyday life. Temporal lobe seizures are also often associated with a feeling of dreaminess or detachment.

- In frontal lobe seizures, there may be uncontrolled jerking or spasm of one arm or leg or the head and eyes may turn to one side.

- In parietal lobe seizures, the patient may experience tingling down one side of the body.

- In occipital lobe seizures, the patient may experience flashing lights in one half of the vision.

  The seizure usually lasts a matter of seconds.

Complex partial seizures

These are really the next stage up from simple partial seizures, and the clue is in the word 'complex'. In these, the seizure involves a larger part of the brain and spreads to enough of the brain so that the patient is no longer aware of his or her environment (that is, becomes unconscious).

The spread of the seizure can either be so fast that the patient does not experience the simple partial seizure, or be slow enough for the patient to have, for example, a feeling of déjà vu, a strange unpleasant taste or an awareness of coloured flashing lights lasting seconds to a few minutes before becoming unaware of the surroundings.

During the seizure, it is quite common for complex, strange or inappropriate actions to occur (called 'automatisms'). For example, the patient may fumble with his or her clothes or make chewing movements. Occasionally, the actions are coordinated and can even take the form of running, dancing, undressing or speaking in a confused fashion.

These seizures usually last a matter of minutes, but are occasionally more prolonged. On coming round, the patient is completely unaware of what he or she has done.

Secondary generalised seizures

These result from the spread of the seizure throughout both halves of the brain; the spread can be slow enough for the patient to have a warning (the aura, which is in fact a simple partial seizure) or so rapid that the patient loses consciousness without an aura.

This spread is called secondary generalisation and the seizure takes the form of a 'generalised tonic–clonic' seizure. In this, the patient often goes stiff (called the tonic phase) and may let out a high-pitched cry; he or she then falls, arms and legs jerk rhythmically (called the clonic phase), and grunting can occur, as can heavy breathing, foaming from the mouth and cyanosis (lips turning blue as a result of lack of oxygen).

During the seizure the patient may bite the tongue or wet him- or herself; it usually lasts a few minutes, and afterwards the patient is often confused, may not know where he or she is and will often sleep. The after-effects (the 'postictal' phase) last for minutes or hours.

This seizure, which used to be called a 'grand mal' attack, is now known as a tonic–clonic seizure, and is also sometimes referred to as a convulsion.

Generalised seizures

These are seizures that begin in both halves of the brain at once; there is no warning and consciousness is lost immediately. Often this seizure is a tonic–clonic seizure (see above), but it can be a clonic seizure (no stiff phase) or a tonic seizure (no shaking stage – the patient just falls like a board). There is also a rare type in which the patient just slumps to the ground, but recovers quite quickly (an atonic seizure).

There are also two other categories of generalised seizures: absences and myoclonic jerks.

Absences

These used to be called a 'petit mal' attack. They are short blank spells, usually in children or young adults. In an absence seizure, the patient freezes and stares, and there is sometimes blinking. The attack lasts just a few seconds, and can be confused with poor attention or loss of concentration.

Children with absence epilepsy can have hundreds of these in a day and often neither the child nor observers are aware of most of them because they are so brief. They are associated with a particular brain wave pattern that is discussed in the next chapter.

Myoclonic seizures

These are usually seen in patients with other seizure types, and are very brief jerks of one limb or the whole body. The patient may describe sudden unsteadiness, lack of coordination or loss of balance. In primary generalised epilepsy these typically occur in the morning in the few hours after awakening.

From this, it can be seen that there are many different types of seizure. There are other conditions that can be mistaken for a seizure and these are discussed in the next chapter.

What causes seizures?
Brain signals
All brain activity depends on the passage of electrical signals. The brain consists of billions of cells called neurons. Each neuron has a cell body and long arms with branches known as axons. It is down these axons that the electrical signals pass, like a telephone signal down a telephone line.

Excitation and inhibition
When the signal reaches the end of the axon, it causes the release of a chemical. This chemical communicates with a nearby neuron body via special 'receivers' called receptors. They may 'excite' this neuron body and, if the excitation is sufficient, then a further signal is sent (or 'fired') down its axon. This is the way in which the neurons communicate with each other.

If only excitation took place in the brain, then eventually all the neurons would be firing together, so causing an 'electrical storm' such as seen in a seizure. But some neurons release a chemical from their axons that inhibits the surrounding neurons, stopping them from 'firing'.

How brain activity travels along nerve cells

Brain activity consists of electrical signals in the nerve cells. Electrical signals are carried along a nerve cell via its axon. For a signal to cross the synapse (gap) between two nerve cells, chemical neurotransmitters must pass from the synaptic knob to receptor cells on the next nerve cell.

Imbalance of excitation and inhibition

The brain functions properly when there is a balance

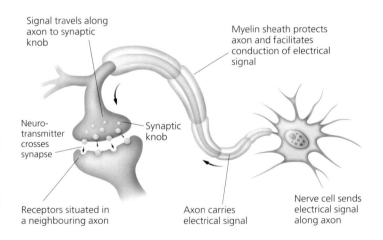

Electrical signals are carried along a nerve cell via its axon. For a signal to cross the synapse (gap) between two nerve cells, chemical neurotransmitters must pass from the synaptic knob to receptor cells on the next cell.

between the excitation and the inhibition. If there is either too much excitation or too little inhibition in a part of the brain (an imbalance), a seizure can result.

Partial seizures

In partial seizures, the local imbalance between excitation and inhibition can be caused by local damage to the brain – for instance, from lack of oxygen at birth, meningitis or head injuries – or by abnormal tissue such as a brain tumour or a defect in brain development. In some cases, the reasons for the partial seizures are not always known.

Generalised seizures

In generalised seizures, the chemical imbalance affects a wide area of brain, and the brain often shows no obviously abnormal structures. This can be caused by drugs, alterations of the body chemistry, excessive alcohol, or inherited or unknown factors.

Thus epileptic seizures are a symptom of an underlying brain disturbance in the same way that stomachache is a symptom of an underlying gut disturbance (for example, food poisoning, ulcers, appendicitis).

When are seizures classed as epilepsy?

Epilepsy is defined as a condition in which the person is prone to recurrent epileptic seizures, so diagnosis is a reflection of the probability of having epileptic seizures.

How likely are you to have another seizure?

If you have one seizure brought on by excessive alcohol, and then you become teetotal, the chances of having another seizure are small and you would not be diagnosed as having epilepsy. If, on the other hand, you had a number of seizures because of a damaged part of your brain, the chances of having another seizure are very high; you would be diagnosed as having epilepsy.

The decision about whether a patient does or does not have epilepsy is not always clear cut. We all have a lifetime chance of having a seizure of about 1 in 30 (29 to 1 against – 'an outside chance'), and we can considerably increase our chances of having a seizure by drinking excessively or taking certain drugs.

Most doctors diagnose patients as having epilepsy only if they have two seizures within a year, because, in this instance, the chances of having a third seizure are probably over 80 per cent (4 to 1 on – 'a sure thing').

The difficulty arises in patients who have had one seizure, and in this instance the doctor usually assesses the chances of another seizure, aided and abetted by various investigations, and by knowledge of the type of seizure and the probable cause. Most doctors in the UK would not usually treat one single seizure as epilepsy because of the low odds of having another seizure (less than 50/50) and the possible side effects of medication.

When can you be declared free of epilepsy?
The second difficult question is, if a patient is diagnosed as having epilepsy, how many seizure-free years must pass before he or she is no longer thought to have epilepsy?

Unfortunately, there is no simple answer to this question, but it is certainly true that most people with epilepsy eventually stop having seizures and thus should not be regarded as having epilepsy (if someone has not had a headache for 10 years, it would be perverse to call him or her a headache sufferer).

Logically a patient stops having epilepsy immediately after the last seizure. How long one has to wait before one can be sure that a seizure was the last will depend on individual circumstances.

It is important to bear in mind that epilepsy is a symptom and not a disease as such. A symptom is something experienced by patients, indicative of an underlying disease. This is the case with epilepsy, which should be considered as an indicator of some underlying brain problem. A wide spectrum of brain conditions can result in epilepsy. Common causes are discussed in the next chapter.

What is an epileptic syndrome?

Sometimes, epilepsy is categorised into syndromes. These categories are particularly useful in children. A syndrome is a medical term referring to a specific condition in which characteristic groups of symptoms occur together.

Syndromes are sometimes named after the person who first described them. For example, West's syndrome consists of infantile spasms (epileptic attacks in which the baby suddenly flexes or stiffens) with a particular brain wave pattern and often mental handicap in babies aged between three and twelve months. Most go on to have epilepsy that is difficult to treat and a learning disorder.

Syndromes can have many causes, although often no cause can be identified. Some syndromes are termed 'idiopathic', which means that they are the result of genetic or constitutional abnormalities (for

Features of epileptic syndromes

Epilepsy occurs in many different forms and some forms are called epileptic syndromes. These are conditions in which certain symptoms occur together. The two most commonly found types of epileptic syndrome are benign childhood epilepsy and primary generalised epilepsy. The chart below lists the distinguishing features of these two syndromes.

Epileptic syndrome	Features
Benign childhood epilepsy with centrotemporal spikes	• Occurs between 2 and 14 years • Can be inherited • Seizures involve face, throat and tongue, and consciousness is preserved • Occasionally tonic–clonic seizures occur during sleep • Typical EEG pattern • Most get completely better and drug treatment is not usually necessary
Primary generalised epilepsy	• Usually occurs in childhood or adolescence • Can be divided into many different subtypes • Can be inherited • Seizure types consist of a combination of absences, tonic–clonic seizures and myoclonic seizures • Seizures usually occur on, or within a couple of hours of, waking • Typical EEG pattern • Usually well controlled with the antiepileptic drug valproate

example, idiopathic generalised epilepsy or benign childhood epilepsy with centrotemporal spikes).

The most common epileptic syndromes are benign childhood epilepsy with centrotemporal spikes (this is a term that refers to the distinctive electroencephalo-graph or EEG changes recorded from the heart) and primary generalised or generalised epilepsies. The box on page 17 outlines the features that characterise these two epileptic syndromes.

KEY POINTS

- Seizures in different parts of the brain produce different effects

- Seizures take many forms and can be likened to electrical storms in the brain

Diagnosis of epilepsy

What does the doctor look for?

When a doctor first sees somebody with possible epilepsy, there are two questions that are addressed:

1 Does the patient definitely have epileptic seizures?

2 What is the cause of the epilepsy?

Is it epilepsy?

Many conditions can be confused with epileptic seizures. In adults, the most common are:

- syncope (fainting)

- migraine

- hyperventilation (over-breathing) and panic attacks

- pseudo-seizures.

In children, other conditions that are also commonly confused with epilepsy include breath-holding attacks and night terrors.

Syncope

Syncope is the medical term for fainting, and occurs when not enough blood gets to the brain. The most common mechanism of syncope is the classic swoon (the 'vasovagal' attack), in response to, for instance, seeing something unpleasant, experiencing excruciating pain or standing for a long period of time in a hot enclosed space.

Occasionally, syncope is the result of a heart disturbance (for example, if the heart goes into an abnormal rhythm) or it can be precipitated by particular events (including coughing or urinating).

The classic faint is well known to all of us; the person feels dizzy, hot and sick, becomes very pale (a deathly white), his or her vision goes grey and then he or she slumps to the ground. At this point, the blood flow to the brain increases and the person comes round quite quickly.

At first sight, it would seem difficult to confuse this with the seizures mentioned in the previous chapter. However, some jerking of the limbs can occur, especially if the person is propped up, because this may prevent enough blood reaching the brain.

The jerking is occasionally prolonged, but seldom has the coordinated pattern of a tonic–clonic seizure. In some partial seizures, the person may experience similar feelings to those of a faint so that the two conditions are not always easy to distinguish.

Migraine

Migraines often begin with a disturbance in vision or can be associated with tingling in the arm or face, and rarely with a disturbance of speech. It can be difficult to distinguish this from a simple partial seizure, especially because it is not uncommon to have a splitting headache after a seizure.

Consciousness is, however, practically never lost with a migraine. There are also differences in the disturbance of vision between that in migraine and that in epilepsy.

Disturbances of vision in migraine usually evolve over minutes, and have a simple form (for example, circles of light or bright dots, or a jagged appearance). Disturbances of vision in epilepsy evolve more rapidly over seconds and are usually more complex (for example, multi-coloured shapes or sometimes scenes and faces).

In addition, if tingling is experienced, it tends to spread slowly up the arm in migraine and rapidly in seizures. In most cases, there is little doubt about whether an attack is caused by migraine or epilepsy, but occasionally it can present a diagnostic puzzle.

Hyperventilation and panic attacks

Over-breathing (hyperventilation) is not uncommon, especially in those under a lot of stress or in those who tend to panic ('panic attacks'). The immediate feeling is usually described as a sudden difficulty in catching one's breath, and a feeling of panic (although these do not always have to be present).

During over-breathing, a person breathes out too much carbon dioxide and when this happens the acidity of the blood changes. This affects nerve activity and can cause tingling sensations, spasms of the hand, light-headedness and even blackouts. These attacks are best treated with relaxation and breathing exercises.

Breathing into a bag during an attack enables a person to re-breathe the carbon dioxide that he or she is breathing out and this prevents or reverses the unpleasant effects of hyperventilation.

'Pseudo-seizures'

These are often the most difficult to distinguish from true epileptic seizures. These attacks are frequently referred to as dissociative seizures or a non-epileptic attack disorder.

These attacks are 'all in the mind', although usually involuntary and occurring without any conscious motivation. Occasionally these attacks are 'put on', but for the most part the patient has little control and they can be likened to an emotional outburst.

The patient may fall, appear to lose consciousness, and then thrash around or lie motionless. These attacks often have some deep-rooted emotional basis, and may require psychiatric and/or psychological treatment. They do not respond to drugs for epilepsy.

When it is difficult to tell these from an epileptic seizure, patients may need to be admitted to hospital for close observation.

Breath-holding attacks

Unfortunately toddlers can hold their breath until they turn blue, and may resort to this if they do not get their own way. Usually the attack stops there, but occasionally strong-willed toddlers can hold their breath until they pass out.

These attacks do not require drug treatment, and usually stop of their own accord.

Night terrors

These usually affect young children, but they can continue into adulthood. A few hours after falling asleep, the child appears to wake, is terrified and cannot be comforted.

In the morning the child usually has no memory of the night's events. Although worrying, these are completely innocent and do not require treatment.

Investigating epilepsy
Medical history
The most important diagnostic tool is the 'medical history' – the question-and-answer session that occurs between patient and doctor in the consulting room or surgery.

The doctor will try to determine whether the episodes are seizures by asking for a detailed description of what happens, and obviously, as consciousness may be impaired, it is important that there is someone present who has seen an episode in order to help with the description (or even better a video of the episode).

The doctor will be interested in what the underlying cause of the seizures is and will thus ask questions about head injuries, problems with birth, whether the patient has had meningitis or consumed alcohol, and whether other people in the family have epilepsy. He or she will also be interested in the impact that epilepsy will have on the patient's life and so will ask about the patient's job and home life.

Medical examination
Last of all, the doctor will examine the patient, looking for clues as to whether there is some underlying brain abnormality, and may also check the heart, especially if syncope is suspected. A detailed neurological examination involves checking the eyes, the face,

coordination, power and sensation in the limbs, and the reflexes in the arms, legs and feet.

Besides blood and other routine tests, there are three special investigations: electroencephalography, computed tomography (CT) and magnetic resonance imaging (MRI). These are described below.

Electroencephalography
How is it done?
Electroencephalography is literally 'recording the electricity from the brain'. Wires are attached to different parts of the head, which are then connected to an amplifier; this amplifier magnifies the small electrical signal from the brain and records this signal into a computer.

An EEG is merely a recording of the internal electrical patterns of the brain, and does not involve the passage of any electricity into or out of the brain. It is thus a harmless and painless investigation, and is of great diagnostic use.

Recording electrical activity in the brain
By attaching small electrodes to the patient's scalp, a doctor can use a machine that measures the electro-encephalogram/-graph (EEG) to monitor brain activity. The patient's brain waves are displayed on the screen. The EEG is helpful in making diagnoses.

Abormal brain waves in epilepsy
Normally, the tracing shows a wave pattern (the 'brain waves') with one wave occurring every tenth of a second or so. The waves slow down during sleep, and speed up when the patient is alert. If the patient is prone to epilepsy, the electrical pattern may be

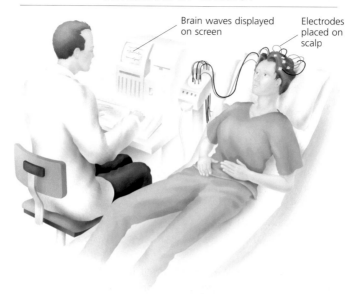

Brain waves displayed on screen

Electrodes placed on scalp

By attaching small electrodes to the patient's scalp, a doctor can use an electroencephalography machine to monitor brain activity. The patient's brain waves are displayed on the screen.

different, and is likely to show what are called spikes or spike/wave patterns.

Spikes can be picked up by an EEG performed in between seizures in only about half the patients with epilepsy, but, if spikes are present, there is a 99 per cent chance that the person has epilepsy. EEGs are occasionally performed during sleep because spikes are more likely to be picked up during this period.

Electrical activity in the brain during epilepsy
The orange trace of this EEG shows the electrical activity in the brain during an epileptic seizure, when a chaotic and unregulated electrical discharge passes through the brain, causing an increase in brain activity.

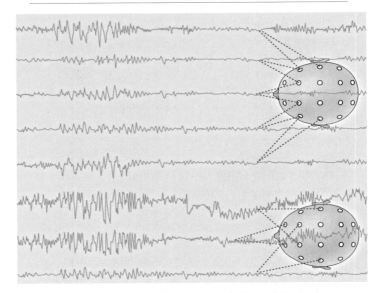

The orange traces of this electroencephalograph (EEG) show the electrical activity in the brain during an epileptic seizure. During an epileptic seizure, a chaotic and unregulated electrical discharge passes through the brain, causing an increase in activity.

What does it tell us?

A particular EEG pattern called three per second spike and wave is of particular importance. This is seen in primary generalised epilepsy, which responds to a specific form of drug treatment and generally has a good outcome.

EEGs performed during a seizure, and especially if the patient is videoed at the same time, are of great use in patients in whom the diagnosis is in some doubt. They also help to identify exactly where the seizure starts (necessary, for instance, in assessing patients for epilepsy surgery).

One such test is called video telemetry. This involves patients being admitted to hospital for several days, during which they are constantly monitored by EEGs and video. Sometimes it is also necessary to reduce or withdraw the patient's antiepileptic drugs to induce a seizure while the patient is being monitored.

Computed tomography
How is it done?
Computed tomography, or CT, is literally the use of a computer to give pictures of 'slices' of the brain. This diagnostic technique uses X-rays.

However, unlike a conventional skull X-ray in which X-rays are fired at one side of the head, with a photographic plate on the other side, in a CT scan X-rays are fired at different angles and picked up by 'receivers' placed all around the head. The information obtained is then analysed by a computer which displays the X-ray signal as a series of pictures of slices through the skull and brain, something like slices through a loaf of bread.

During a CT scan the patient has to lie with his or her head stationary in the scanner for a number of minutes. This is an entirely painless procedure.

Using computed tomography to create a picture of the brain
The patient lies with his or her head in a scanner while the machine fires X-rays through the brain at different angles. The X-rays are picked up by receivers and the information analysed by a computer to create a picture of the brain.

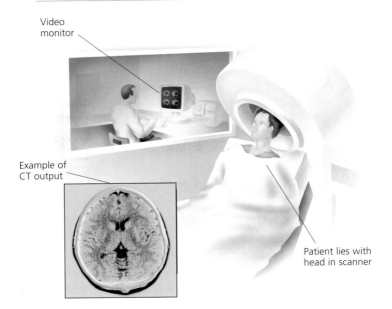

Video monitor

Example of CT output

Patient lies with head in scanner

Computed tomography (CT) fires X-rays through the brain at different angles. The X-rays are picked up by receivers and the information analysed by a computer to create a picture of the brain.

What does it tell us?

By using this technique, it is possible to demonstrate such brain abnormalities as tumours, strokes or brain haemorrhages.

Occasionally a dye is injected into a vein in the arm to highlight certain parts of the brain, in order to gain more information from the scan.

Magnetic resonance imaging

How is it done?

Magnetic resonance imaging (MRI) is a form of brain scan that does not use X-rays at all. A large, powerful magnet is placed around the patient's head. The atoms in the brain line themselves up along this magnetic field.

A burst of radio waves is then 'fired' at the patient and the hydrogen atoms in the brain wobble (resonate). As the hydrogen atoms gradually return to rest, they give off radio waves that are picked up by 'receivers' and analysed by a computer; this gives detailed pictures of the brain.

This technique is very safe and entirely painless; however, it does involve lying in the scanner, which is an enclosed space, for some time (usually 10 to 20 minutes); some people find this unpleasant. Also, because powerful magnets are used, people with some

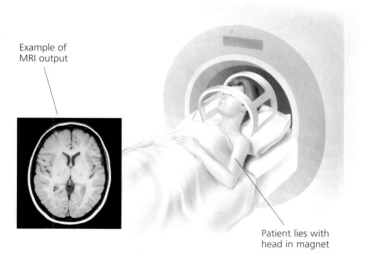

Example of
MRI output

Patient lies with
head in magnet

Magnetic resonance imaging (MRI) can detect many subtle and small abnormalities that are invisible to CT scanning.

types of metal implants (for instance, clips or wires from previous brain or other operations and pacemakers) cannot be scanned.

Using MRI to create a picture of the brain

The patient lies with his or her head surrounded by a large magnet while a burst of radio waves is fired at the brain. The radio waves given off by the brain in response are picked up by receivers and the information analysed by a computer to create a picture of the brain.

What can it tell us?

This technique can detect many subtle and small abnormalities that are invisible to CT. As MRI techniques improve, so the underlying cause of epilepsy is being discovered in more and more patients. MRI is especially useful in assessing the suitability of patients who have not responded to drugs for surgical treatment (see page 55).

Also, using computer analysis, the relative size of different brain structures can be calculated. This is important in, for instance, analysing certain areas of the brain (especially an area known as the hippocampus) which, when damaged, can cause seizures.

Causes of epilepsy

As has been emphasised, epilepsy is a symptom and not a disease. There are many causes such as infections, head injuries, brain tumours, brain injuries at birth and inherited diseases (see the box). Occasionally epilepsy can start many years after the damage has occurred. For many sufferers (over 50 per cent), no known cause is found.

Causes of epilepsy from birth to old age

Often the cause of a person's epilepsy is not known. This chart lists the probable causes of epilepsy in both children and adults. Birth trauma and genetic disease may cause childhood epilepsy, whereas in adults brain tumours or strokes are common causes.

- Inherited brain diseases, for example, tuberous sclerosis

- Inherited epilepsies, for example, primary generalised epilepsy

- Birth trauma

- Convulsions caused by fever (febrile convulsions)

- Brain infections, for example, meningitis, encephalitis, brain abscesses

- Recreational drugs and alcohol, for example, cocaine, amphetamines, ecstasy or 'E'

- Head trauma

- Blood chemical abnormalities, for example, low calcium, magnesium or glucose

- Brain haemorrhage (cerebral haemorrhage)

- Brain tumours, for example, gliomas, meningiomas

- Stroke

- Previous brain surgery

- Dementia, for example, Alzheimer's disease

In the generalised epilepsies, genetic factors are likely to play a role, some epilepsies being hereditary, but in most cases this is not so (how do you inherit a head injury?). Except in a few genetically inherited conditions that can cause epilepsy, the risks of passing the epilepsy on to offspring are very small.

KEY POINTS

■ Many conditions are confused with epilepsy, the most common being fainting, migraine, panic attacks, 'pseudo-seizures', breath-holding attacks and night terrors (the last two in children)

■ Epilepsy can be caused by infections, head injuries, brain tumours, brain injuries at birth and inherited diseases, but often the cause is not known

■ Investigations for diagnosing epilepsy include electroencephalography, CT and MRI, but the 'history' is of the greatest importance in making the diagnosis

■ The risks of passing epilepsy on to offspring are very small

Treatment of epilepsy

Avoiding harm and reducing the number of attacks

Much can be done to prevent a person coming to any great harm during an epileptic attack by following a few simple procedures. Drug therapy can help to cut down on the number of such attacks.

Managing a convulsion

Convulsions are often frightening to watch. The person may turn blue, have wild, jerking movements, foam at the mouth and cry out.

Advice to bystanders

People often wish to intervene by placing an object in the person's mouth to 'prevent him swallowing his tongue' and by calling an ambulance. Placing an object in the mouth can, however, be dangerous because the patient may bite the hand of the helper or bite the object, resulting in damage to the teeth and mouth.

If the person has regular attacks, having an ambulance called every time is embarrassing and usually unnecessary. The box on page 36 shows the correct procedure to follow in the event of a seizure.

Advice to carers

Some patients have recurrent prolonged seizures, and occasionally carers will be asked to give these patients a drug called diazepam either by mouth or as a suppository in order to stop or prevent the seizure. This policy should be discussed with the doctor in charge of the care of any patient who has repeated episodes of seizures lasting longer than 20 to 30 minutes, because immediate drug therapy may terminate the attack and prevent the patient needing to go to hospital.

The recovery position

Once a convulsion is over, the patient should be put into the recovery position. The pictures on page 37 show how to move someone into the position with least strain to the patient or yourself.

Long-term treatment

The aim of long-term treatment is to stop all seizures, and this can be attained in most (about 80 per cent) patients. The following are the three main ways to achieve this:

1 Avoiding factors that provoke seizures

2 Drug treatment

3 Brain surgery.

Very occasionally, patients who have warnings that last a long time before losing consciousness are able to

What to do during a convulsion

It can be dangerous to place an object in the mouth of someone having a seizure and it is usually unnecessary to call an ambulance. There are a few simple procedures that should be followed by an onlooker during a seizure and these are listed below. The most important thing is to stay calm and let the seizure run its course.

- During a convulsion the patient should be laid on the ground away from objects that can cause injury, the head should be cushioned and the patient should not be restrained in any way. No attempt should be made to put anything in the mouth in the mistaken belief that this may prevent the person biting the tongue.

- After the convulsion, the patient should be turned on to their left side, in the recovery position (see next page), and someone should remain with the patient until he or she is fully recovered.

- Sometimes, confusion can mimic aggression. In these cases the patient should not be restrained, but gently coaxed out of danger. At this stage, if anything is blocking the airway, it should be cleared.

- If the convulsion lasts longer than five minutes, or if the patient is having repeated convulsions without consciousness being regained in between attacks, then an ambulance should be called.

The recovery position

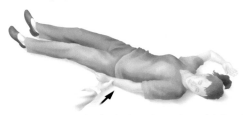

1. With the patient lying on her back place the patient's left hand to the side of her body. Turn the head to the left.

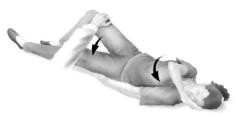

2. Tuck the patient's right hand under the left side of the face and jaw. Bend the patient's right leg at the knee and then pull the patient gently over to her left by the right knee and right shoulder so she is resting on her left side.

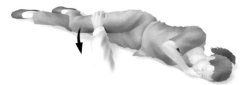

3. Raise the right leg at the hip while keeping the knee bent. Ensure that the left arm is behind the body, not underneath. This will stabilise the patient on her left side.

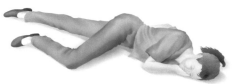

4. The 'recovery position' is complete.

control their seizure and prevent the loss of consciousness. This is achieved by intense concentration during the warning period or by other individually learned methods.

Avoiding factors that provoke seizures

In many patients, avoiding certain factors will lessen the frequency of seizures and in a few will prevent them altogether. Very rarely, people can have seizures brought on by hearing particular pieces of music, reading, hot showers, seeing certain patterns, etc. and these are referred to as 'reflex epilepsies'. For most, however, no specific trigger is ever noticed.

There are nevertheless four things that can induce or worsen seizures in many:

1 excessive alcohol

2 lack of sleep

3 stress

4 fever.

In addition, a few patients are sensitive to flashing lights (this is called photosensitivity – see below).

Seizures can also be minimised by paying attention to general lifestyle issues such as healthy diet, exercise, and attention to psychological and physical well-being.

Alcohol and sleep deprivation

Often patients with primary generalised epilepsies are particularly susceptible to seizures after binges of alcohol or sleep deprivation, so these are almost certainly two factors that all people with epilepsy should try to avoid.

Indeed, chronic alcoholism or binge drinking can frequently induce seizures, and seizures are thus a common complication of alcoholism. For those whose seizures are particularly exacerbated by sleep deprivation, getting tired, missing sleep and sometimes shift work are inadvisable.

Stress

Although it is often difficult to identify the effects of stress, it can nevertheless have a profound effect on seizure control.

Relaxation exercises, stress management and such therapies as aromatherapy can have a beneficial effect, and thus should be recommended to some patients. Often, counselling those who have difficulties coping with their epilepsy can help seizure control.

Depression, low mood and low morale can also increase the frequency of seizures. These factors can also affect how regularly patients take their medication (compliance), and thus indirectly worsen seizure control.

Fever and high temperatures

During any illness seizures can get worse, and this is especially so in young children if a fever is present. Thus, at the first signs of a fever, the body temperature should be kept down with regular paracetamol and, if necessary, a fan.

Another instance in which the body temperature can rise, resulting in increased seizure frequency, is sunstroke, which is usually the result of a combination of excessive sun exposure and dehydration.

Photosensitivity

Many people often have concerns about light sensitivity (photosensitivity) and the relationship of seizures to video games, and television or computer screens. In fact, less than five per cent of all people with epilepsy are sensitive to flashing lights.

The photosensitive seizures usually occur with lights that flicker from 5 to 30 times per second so television and video games (both of which have flickering screens) can induce photosensitive seizures in susceptible individuals. However, children in the UK spend a large amount of time watching television and playing video games, and thus any seizure that occurs during this time may be purely coincidental. It should be emphasised that the great majority of people with epilepsy can quite safely watch TV and video screens.

Other common precipitants of photosensitive seizures include:

- sunlight reflecting off water

- passing a line of trees through which the sun is shining

- stroboscopic lights (although local authorities do have guidelines on the flash rate of strobe lighting, these are perhaps best avoided by susceptible individuals).

In some patients with photosensitivity, avoidance of what triggers their seizures or taking certain precautions, such as the use of sunglasses in bright light, rather than antiepileptic drug treatment, may be all that they need to do to prevent the seizures.

The following are the precautions that can be taken to avoid television-induced seizures for those not on drugs:

- Viewing the television in a well-lit room

- Viewing the television from an angle

- Sitting at least 2.5 metres from the television set

- Changing channels with a remote control rather than getting too close to the screen

- Covering one eye

- Using high-frequency (100 Hz) televisions.

Seizures are rarely triggered by watching a film at a cinema, and computer screens usually operate at a sufficiently high frequency to avoid provoking seizures. However, in both these instances, if the content consists of a changing geometric pattern at a certain frequency, it can very occasionally provoke a seizure.

Antiepileptic drug treatment is usually effective in preventing photosensitive seizures.

Drug treatment

Since the earliest times, people have been seeking effective drugs for epilepsy, and through the ages such cures as powdered human skull, vultures' blood and mistletoe have all been tried.

The first effective therapy, however, was reported in 1857 by Sir Charles Locock, an obstetrician, who had an interest in epilepsy because of the mistaken idea, common at that time, that in some women epilepsy came from their wombs. The drug he used was potassium bromide, which was the most effective therapy until 1912 when phenobarbital (or phenobarbitone as it was then known) was introduced.

The main problems with bromides are their unacceptable side effects. In fact the trade-off between side effects and effectiveness of an antiepileptic drug is still at the heart of antiepileptic drug treatment.

Absorbing the dose

Once swallowed, an antiepileptic drug is absorbed into the bloodstream, passing into the brain which is where the drug acts. Whether an antiepileptic drug is taken on an empty or a full stomach can affect the amount of drug absorbed. In general they should be taken at the same time in relation to meals.

Once the drug has passed around the bloodstream it is removed from the body, either being broken down (metabolised) by the liver or filtered out by the kidneys and passed out in the urine (different drugs are removed in different ways).

If a drug is removed from the body very quickly, then it has to be taken frequently (three to four times a day) to keep the blood levels reasonably high. If a drug is only slowly removed then it can be taken once a day.

How antiepileptic drugs are used by the body

Once swallowed, antiepileptic drugs enter the bloodstream from the digestive system. They travel to the brain where they can have a beneficial effect. When they reach the liver, they are broken down and the waste product is taken out of the blood by the kidneys. This then passes out of the body in the urine.

How do these drugs work?

It is not certain exactly how most antiepileptic drugs work, but there do seem to be a number of important mechanisms. In an earlier chapter (see page 12),

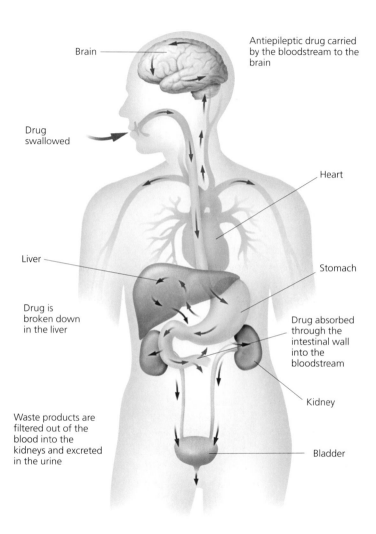

Brain

Antiepileptic drug carried
by the bloodstream to the
brain

Drug
swallowed

Heart

Liver

Stomach

Drug is
broken down
in the liver

Drug absorbed
through the
intestinal wall
into the
bloodstream

Kidney

Waste products are
filtered out of the
blood into the
kidneys and excreted
in the urine

Bladder

How antiepileptic drugs are used by the body.

it was explained that seizures may result when the excitation and inhibition occurring in the brain are not balanced.

Some antiepileptic drugs correct this chemical imbalance. Other antiepileptic drugs 'stabilise' neurons, and thus prevent excessive firing of axons.

Choosing the right drug

The art of treatment is to choose the drug that suits the patient best. What is a very effective drug in one patient may be useless in another, and different drugs are more or less effective in different patient profiles.

Some antiepileptic drugs act only in some types of epilepsy (for example, ethosuximide in absence seizures), and indeed some drugs can make some forms of epilepsy worse (for example, carbamazepine in myoclonic seizures). A list of the drugs that are used most often in particular seizure types is presented in the box opposite.

Side effects

There are three main types of side effects of antiepileptic drugs:

1 Dose related

2 Individual or idiosyncratic

3 Chronic.

Dose-related side effects

These are seen in all patients if the dose of the antiepileptic drug is high enough (this is sometimes called drug intoxication). The amount of drug that can be tolerated varies from patient to patient.

Types of seizure and appropriate drug treatments

For effective treatment a drug has to be chosen from the large number that are available. Some anticonvulsant drugs work only for particular forms of epilepsy. It is important to choose the right drug to suit the patient and the type of seizures being experienced. The chart below shows the main drugs that are chosen for particular types of epilepsy.

Seizure type	Drugs used		
Partial seizures			
Simple partial	Acetazolamide	Levetiracetam	Primidone
Complex partial	Carbamazepine	Oxcarbazepine	Tiagabine
Secondary	Clobazam	Phenobarbital	Topiramate
generalised	Gabapentin	Phenytoin	Valproate
	Lamotrigine	Pregabalin	Vigabatrin
Generalised seizures			
Absences	Acetazolamide	Ethosuximide	Valproate
	Clobazam	Lamotrigine	
	Clonazepam	Topiramate	
Atonic/tonic	Acetazolamide	Oxcarbazepine	Topiramate
	Carbamazepine	Phenobarbital	Valproate
	Clobazam	Phenytoin	
	Lamotrigine	Primidone	
Tonic–clonic/ clonic	Acetazolamide	Levetiracetam	Topiramate
	Carbamazepine	Oxcarbazepine	Valproate
	Clobazam	Phenobarbital	
	Clonazepam	Phenytoin	
	Lamotrigine	Primidone	
Myoclonic	Acetazolamide	Levetiracetam	Primidone
	Clobazam	Phenobarbital	Valproate
	Clonazepam	Piracetam	

With most of the antiepileptic drugs, dizziness, double vision, unsteadiness, drowsiness and headache are the most common dose-related side effects. They are alleviated by reducing the dose of the drug, but, in the case of drugs that are removed slowly from the body, it may take several days for the effects of dose reduction to be felt.

Importantly some immediate side effects (especially drowsiness) diminish over a few days or weeks, and thus it is always prudent to take a drug for a month or so before abandoning it because of mild side effects. Most of the antiepileptic drugs can also interfere with concentration and intellectual ability.

Idiosyncratic side effects

These are usually allergic reactions. They take the form of rashes or various blood disorders. As they do not depend on drug dosage, the only way to overcome these side effects is to discontinue the particular drug.

Chronic side effects

These are the ones that occur after taking the drug for months or years. The chronic side effects of the newer antiepileptic drugs are thus not as well documented as the chronic side effects of the older, more established drugs. The box on page 47 includes the more common side effects that can occur with some antiepileptic drugs.

There is some evidence that long-term use of certain antiepileptic drugs is associated with thinning of the bones (osteoporosis) – a condition that can increase the risk of fractures.

Possible side effects of antiepileptic drugs

Antiepileptic drugs can produce three main types of side effect: dose related, individual or chronic. Dose-related side effects are dependent on drug dose, individual or idiosyncratic side effects are rare allergic reactions and chronic side effects are those seen in long-term treatment.

Dose related	Idiosyncratic	Chronic
Double vision	Rash	Weight gain
Unsteadiness	Blood disorders	Vitamin
Dizziness	Liver failure	deficiencies
Sleepiness	Psychosis/	Cosmetic
Headache	depression	changes
Stomach upset		Acne
Slowness		Mood changes
		Osteoporosis

Drug interactions

The blood levels of antiepileptic drugs can be affected by other drugs (including other antiepileptic drugs), resulting in either a fall in the blood level (causing seizures) or a rise in the blood level (causing side effects). This is because the breakdown, excretion and absorption of antiepileptic drugs can be affected by other drugs.

It is thus important to check before taking any other medication, including those that can be bought without a prescription (see box on page 49 for some of the commonly prescribed drugs that can interact with some antiepileptic drugs). When a new antiepileptic drug is added to a patient's antiepileptic drug treatment, it is often necessary to change the dose of the existing antiepileptic drugs and to monitor blood levels.

The introduction of an oral contraceptive can substantially alter the levels of some antiepileptic drugs, sometimes necessitating a major change in dose. An example is the interaction of lamotrigine and the contraceptive pill.

Antiepileptic drugs can also affect the blood levels of other drugs. Two important examples are interaction with the oral contraceptive and interaction with warfarin.

The former may result in a faster rate of metabolism of the contraceptive, rendering it ineffective. If this happens, higher doses of the pill are required. Breakthrough bleeding (between menstrual periods) is a sign that the dose of the pill is probably not high enough, and that it will not be providing adequate contraception.

A similar increase in drug metabolism occurs when antiepileptic drugs are combined with warfarin (a drug for preventing blood clotting), and this may result in the need for larger doses of warfarin.

Starting and stopping antiepileptic drugs

Starting antiepileptic drugs at a high dose can result in side effects. Antiepileptic drugs should therefore be introduced cautiously and the dose increased in gradual steps.

The final dose is determined by the balance between seizure control and side effects. It is important to realise that individual patients require different doses and that the final dose may be even more than the generally recommended maximum dose for the drug.

Examples of medications that interact with antiepileptic drugs

As with all medications, taking one can affect the activity of another. Below are examples of commonly prescribed medications that interact with antiepileptic drugs.

Medication	Treatment use
Allopurinol	Gout
Aminophylline	Asthma
Amiodarone	Heart rhythm disturbances
Antacids	Indigestion
Aspirin	Pain-killer
Cimetidine	Indigestion, peptic ulcers
Co-proxamol	Pain-killer
Co-trimoxazole	Antibiotic
Diltiazem	Angina
Erythromycin	Antibiotic
Fluoxetine	Antidepressant
Folic acid	Vitamin
Haloperidol	Antipsychotic
Imipramine	Antidepressant
Omeprazole	Indigestion, peptic ulcers
Verapamil	Angina

Antiepileptic drugs that can interfere with the contraceptive pill

Oral contraceptives are particularly prone to interacting with antiepileptic drugs. The antiepileptic drugs with which they interfere are:

carbamazepine   lamotrigine   oxcarbazepine
phenobarbital   phenytoin   primidone
topiramate

In this instance, there is usually no need for concern if the patient is not experiencing side effects. If a drug does not work or if the side effects are unacceptable another drug is tried.

Most patients are controlled on only one antiepileptic drug (monotherapy – literally one therapy). In a smaller number of patients, two or more different antiepileptic drugs are necessary (this is called polytherapy – literally many therapies).

For the following reasons the doctor will try, wherever possible, to avoid polytherapy:

- Some antiepileptic drugs interact with other antiepileptic drugs.

- Side effects are often greater in polytherapy.

- It is difficult to remember to take many different drugs and thus compliance (see below) is worse.

- There is a greater potential for mistakes.

Stopping antiepileptic drugs

When a drug is being stopped, the dose must be decreased in gradual steps. A flurry of severe seizures can result from stopping an antiepileptic drug suddenly, even if the drug had not apparently been effective.

Taking drugs regularly

The taking of a drug according to instructions received is known as compliance. Poor compliance (that is, failure to take a drug as instructed – either not taking the drug at all or taking it irregularly) is a major cause of failure of antiepileptic drug treatment.

As it usually takes some time (days or weeks) for an antiepileptic drug to be fully effective, and seizure occurrence is usually unpredictable, it is imperative to take the drug regularly in order to prevent seizures. When patients are not having seizures, they feel perfectly well (apart from the side effects of the antiepileptic drugs), and so it is thus not surprising that the occasional dose is missed either consciously or subconsciously.

Regular routine
It is also very easy for patients on regular medication to forget whether or not the last dose was taken. It is important for patients to build up a regular routine of drug taking.

Compliance is not helped if a drug has to be taken more than twice a day, especially in children who are not keen to take drugs midday at school. The situation becomes even worse if the patient is on polytherapy.

A drug wallet, with the tablets divided into different compartments according to the time of day and the day of the week, is often very useful. All that then needs to be done is for the compartments in the wallet to be replenished each week. Drug wallets are also useful for those who have poor memories or very busy routines.

A drug wallet can help compliance
There are many types of drug organiser available to suit different needs. The one shown on page 52 is a drug wallet. A drug organiser can help you to take the right pill at the right time of day.

Stopping suddenly
Occasionally, patients decide to stop their drugs suddenly (often because of depression or low morale).

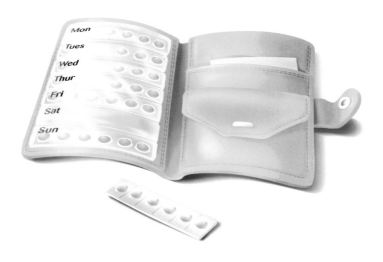

A medication organiser will help you to take the right pill at the right time of day.

This is potentially dangerous and can lead to prolonged and frequent seizures.

Also, during periods of vomiting or diarrhoea, the tablets may not be absorbed, and in these cases the tablets should be retaken or anti-sickness (antiemetic) drugs prescribed by the doctor. On occasion admission to hospital is necessary.

Taking the right dose

Last of all, misunderstandings between doctors and patients can lead to the wrong dosages being taken. After any consultation with the doctor, it is important to be clear precisely about the dose of each drug that should be taken. If necessary the doctor should write this information down.

When coming for appointments, it is usually a good idea for patients to bring their drugs with them. Answers to vague enquiries about drugs are rarely helpful – for example, it would be impossible to give a response to 'Well, I take two blue or is it red pills in the morning, and then a white. No, I take the white pill in the evening'.

Monitoring antiepileptic drugs

It is important to monitor the effectiveness of an antiepileptic drug, and the best method is by seizure frequency. It is often surprisingly difficult to remember exactly how many seizures have occurred and thus a written record (seizure diary) is mandatory for most patients.

Seizure diary

The seizure diary can then be reviewed at each appointment with the doctor. It is important for patients to learn to differentiate between their different seizure types, and to record the frequency of each of them separately. Information about when antiepileptic drugs were started should also be included.

Blood samples

The most important guide to dosage is how well the seizures are controlled and whether or not side effects occur. However, occasionally it is helpful to take a blood sample (usually before the morning dose, although this is not always practical) in order to work out the blood levels of an antiepileptic drug.

Taking a blood sample

Occasionally it is helpful to take a blood sample in

order to ascertain the blood levels of an antiepileptic drug. A fine needle is inserted into a vein in the arm and a small sample withdrawn.

Much is made of blood levels, but it is important to keep these in context. The levels at which most patients have good seizure control with few side effects give rise to the so-called 'therapeutic range' of blood levels for some antiepileptic drugs.

The problem is that we are all individuals and what is an effective blood level for most people may be too high or too low for a minority. Blood levels can, however, give the doctor a rough idea of whether the dose of a drug is adequate.

There are also other circumstances in which blood levels are very useful:

- If seizures are poorly controlled (blood levels may have fallen)

- To check for compliance

- If other drugs (including other antiepileptic drugs) that can interfere with the antiepileptic drug therapy are started

- During pregnancy and illness when drug levels may change

- In patients with severe learning difficulties who may not be able to communicate whether or not they are experiencing side effects.

The next chapter describes the various drugs available for treatment of epilepsy individually.

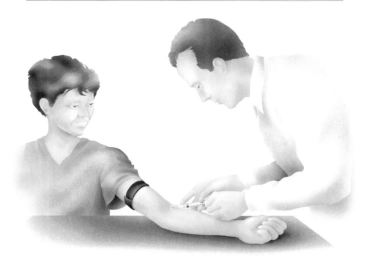

Occasionally it is helpful to take a blood sample in order to ascertain the blood levels of an antiepileptic drug.

Surgery for epilepsy

It has been estimated that about 12,500 patients with epilepsy in the UK could benefit from epilepsy surgery. The potential for and the success of surgery may increase as the technique called magnetic resonance imaging (MRI – see pages 28–30) improves and the cause of seizures can be identified in more and more patients.

Epilepsy surgery is a major undertaking, because it involves removing the part of the brain where the seizures begin and obviously this is not without risk. Epilepsy surgery is therefore reserved for those patients with seizures resistant to drug treatment (also known as 'drug-resistant', 'refractory' or 'pharmacoresistant' patients) and in whom there is little chance of the seizures improving.

Who should have surgery?

Even before investigating patients for epilepsy surgery, several other criteria have to be fulfilled:

- It has to be felt that the seizures are one of the main causes of a patient's disability (a severely handicapped patient may have uncontrolled seizures that are only a minor problem compared with the rest of his or her disability).

- Similarly, it has to be felt by both the doctor and the patient that stopping the seizures would result in a significant improvement in the quality of life. Undertaking brain surgery in someone who is suicidal or severely depressed for reasons other than their epilepsy or in whom the epilepsy is only of small consequence is obviously not to be recommended.

- The patient must be able to understand the possible risks and benefits of the epilepsy surgery.

Tests before surgery

There are several tests that have to be performed:

- Brain imaging by MRI is used in order to identify brain abnormalities that may be the cause of the epilepsy. If no such abnormality can be detected, this does not preclude epilepsy surgery, but makes it considerably less likely to be successful and rarely worth pursuing.

- Psychological testing is carried out in some detail. This involves a number of word tests, memory tests and drawing/constructing tests that elucidate the functioning of different parts of a person's brain.

This kind of testing is performed in order to identify whether any psychological problem or condition present is related to the part of the brain causing the seizures, the importance of this part of the brain for a patient's memory, speech, etc., and last as a baseline for comparison with psychology after the surgery.

- The measurement of the brain waves by electroencephalography also plays a pivotal role. Usually this involves a technique in which the brain waves are correlated with a video of the seizure in order to identify where the seizure starts. This is necessary to check that the abnormality seen on MRI correlates with the part of the brain producing the seizures.

- A test called the sodium amytal test is also sometimes carried out. This involves injecting the anaesthetic agent, sodium amytal, into each side of the brain in turn; the injection is through a tube inserted into the main blood vessel in the groin and then passed up to the blood vessels supplying the brain.

  It is a relatively painless and safe procedure. As a result of the injection, each half of the brain is anaesthetised in turn for a few minutes. During this period, the patient's memory and ability to name objects are tested. Failure to complete the tests accurately means that the half of the brain anaesthetised controls language and memory.

- In most people language resides in the left half of the brain and memory in both, but in a few people this pattern is lost. This is important to know, because the effects of brain surgery on speech, understanding and memory are vital factors in deciding whether surgery is indicated and what type of operation is possible.

- Last, it is common for a psychiatric assessment to be performed in order to confirm that there is no mental illness present which would prevent the patient from having brain surgery (for example, very severe depression) and which needs to be treated before surgery is performed.

When all this information is available, the patient's hospital doctors and the brain surgeon meet to discuss the risks and benefits of epilepsy surgery for each individual patient. Once this has been decided, the risks and the likely benefits are put to the patient who then has to make a decision whether or not to proceed to surgery.

How effective is surgery?

The outcome for epilepsy surgery depends largely on the type of operation, the part of the brain involved and the underlying cause of the epilepsy.

In patients with an identifiable defect in the temporal lobe of the brain (the most common situation), about 70 per cent will become seizure free after surgery, and another 20 per cent will have some improvement.

This does, however, still leave one patient in 10 who has no improvement or who may be worse. Nevertheless, with improved imaging and surgical techniques, the outcome of epilepsy surgery continues to improve.

Vagal nerve stimulation

In some patients, who have drug-resistant epilepsy but are not suitable for brain surgery, vagal nerve stimulation is a possible treatment. This involves the repetitive electrical stimulation of a nerve in the neck (the vagus nerve).

A small operation

The patient undergoes a small operation in which a stimulator (a small box much like a pacemaker) is placed under the skin of the upper chest and a wire from the stimulator is tunnelled to the neck, where it is wrapped around the vagus nerve. After the operation, the stimulator is switched on, and it generates repeated short electrical stimulations.

The intensity, length and frequency of these stimulations can be adjusted by a specialist using a computer that communicates with the stimulator. In addition, patients who have warnings of seizures can activate the stimulator using a magnet. Every five to ten years, the battery of the stimulator needs to be replaced in a further minor operation.

How effective is it?

Vagal nerve stimulation rarely results in the person becoming seizure free, but it offers about a 50 per cent chance of greatly improving seizures. The side effects are usually mild and consist of throat pain and a hoarse voice; these can usually be controlled by adjustment of the stimulation intensity.

This treatment is not more effective than trying a new antiepileptic drug, but can be useful for those who have exhausted all other therapies or who tolerate drugs poorly.

KEY POINTS

- The aim of long-term treatment of epilepsy is to stop seizures

- An antiepileptic drug is chosen to suit the patient

- Side effects of drugs can be dose related, occur in only some individuals or occur only in the long term

- Some patients with epilepsy benefit from brain surgery

Drugs used in the treatment of epilepsy

What can drugs do to help epilepsy?

Most people who experience epileptic seizures find that their symptoms can be controlled with anticonvulsant drug therapy. Some drugs have been around for many years, but others are much more recent.

Established drugs

Some of the most commonly used drugs have been in use since the early part of the twentieth century.

Carbamazepine

This drug has been around since the 1950s, and has been found to be both safe and effective in partial epilepsy and tonic–clonic seizures. It can, however, worsen absences and myoclonic jerks.

Occasionally, a rash or abnormalities of blood counts can occur, which may mean that the drug has to be stopped. Too high a dose can lead to double vision, nausea, headache and drowsiness.

Carbamazepine is also available as a slow-release preparation (once swallowed, the drug is only slowly released from the tablet), which can be taken less frequently and has fewer side effects.

Clonazepam

This drug is one of a group of drugs called benzodiazepines (others are mentioned later), which are better known for their use in anxiety and as sleeping tablets. This drug is effective in absence seizures and other forms of epilepsy. However, in some patients the drug ceases to be effective after a period of time (usually about three months). This phenomenon is called tolerance.

Like all benzodiazepines, drowsiness and behavioural changes (especially aggression in children) are the main side effects.

Ethosuximide

This drug is useful only in absence seizures. Some patients develop a rash, and side effects include stomachache, tiredness, headache and dizziness.

Phenobarbital

This is one of the oldest established antiepileptic drugs, having been used since 1912. It is cheap and effective in most types of epilepsy, but in recent years it has grown out of favour as a result of its side effects. Until recently it was known as phenobarbitone.

Originally, phenobarbital was used as a sleeping pill. It is thus not surprising that some people become drowsy, although this drowsiness is slight and usually improves with time. Paradoxically, it can have the opposite effect in children, and make them hyperactive and aggressive.

In a few, phenobarbital can cause a rash and blistering. Too high a dose leads to drowsiness, impotence, depression and poor memory. With long-term use, phenobarbital can coarsen facial features and decrease the body's stores of certain vitamins (folic acid and vitamin D).

Phenytoin

This drug has been in common usage since 1938. It was initially seen as a breakthrough because it was as effective as phenobarbital but caused less drowsiness. Phenytoin is effective in partial seizures and tonic–clonic seizures.

Some patients get a rash, in which case it should be stopped. Too high a dose can lead to dizziness, increased seizures, drowsiness, unsteadiness and double vision.

Long-term use can lead to swelling of the gums, coarsening of facial features, acne, facial hair and a decrease in the body's stores of certain vitamins (folic acid and vitamin D). As a result of these long-term side effects, young people are not keen to use phenytoin and often a different antiepileptic drug is preferred.

Primidone

This drug is broken down in the body to phenobarbital, and thus has the same side effects and uses as phenobarbital.

Valproate

In France in the 1960s, this drug was discovered to be

useful in epilepsy purely by chance. It is now one of the drugs of choice for light-sensitive (photosensitive) epilepsy, myoclonic seizures and absences. It is, however, effective in all types of epilepsy.

It needs to be used cautiously in children under the age of three years, when it very occasionally causes severe liver damage. Some people can get a drop in the number of platelets in the blood (these are necessary for blood clotting). There have been recent concerns that valproate may be one of the less safe antiepileptic drugs to take during pregnancy.

The most common side effects, however, are stomach upset, hair loss, menstrual irregularities, tremor, swelling of the ankles, weight gain and drowsiness (especially if given with phenobarbital). Valproate is available as a slow-release preparation.

The most common side effects, however, are stomach upset, hair loss, menstrual irregularities, tremor, swelling of the ankles, weight gain and drowsiness (especially if given with phenobarbital). Valproate and carbamazepine are available as slow-release preparations.

The newer drugs

When new antiepileptic drugs are first developed, they are tried on patients with uncontrolled epilepsy (usually partial epilepsy), as add-on therapy to existing antiepileptic drug courses. If they prove to be successful, then initially they are licensed just for this purpose.

Some new antiepileptic drugs are, however, effective in types of epilepsy that fall outside the scope of the licence, and doctors are permitted to prescribe drugs for such conditions, but usually discuss this with the patient

Antiepileptic drugs and their year of introduction in the UK

Some antiepileptic drugs have been in use for a long time, others have only recently been introduced. Below is a list of the drugs with their trade name in brackets and the year that they were first used in the UK.

Scientific or generic name (trade or proprietary name)	Year of introduction
Phenobarbital/phenobarbitone	1912
Phenytoin (Epanutin)	1938
Primidone (Mysoline)	1952
Ethosuximide (Zarontin)	1960
Carbamazepine (Tegretol)	1963
Diazepam (Valium)	1973
Clonazepam (Rivotril)	1974
Valproate (Epilim)	1974
Clobazam (Frisium)	1982
Vigabatrin (Sabril)	1989
Slow-release carbamazepine (Tegretol Retard)	1989
Lamotrigine (Lamictal)	1991
Gabapentin (Neurontin)	1993
Slow-release valproate (Epilim Chrono)	1993
Topiramate (Topamax)	1995
Tiagabine (Gabitril)	1998
Fosphenytoin (Pro-Epanutin)	1998
Levetiracetam (Keppra)	2000
Oxcarbazepine (Trileptal)	2000
Pregabalin (Lyrica)	2004
Zonisamide (Zonegran)	2005

first. Some of these drugs offer advantages over certain older drugs, as they may have fewer side effects.

Gabapentin

At present, gabapentin is licensed to be used only in partial epilepsy in combination with other antiepileptic drugs. It has few side effects, but at higher doses can cause dizziness, tremor and drowsiness; the frequency of seizures can also increase in some patients. The drug can result in weight gain.

Lamotrigine

This drug originally had the same restricted licence as gabapentin, but can now be used as monotherapy. It is potentially useful in most types of epilepsy.

In a few patients, it causes a rash and this seems to be more likely to occur if a patient is started at too high a dose, which causes drowsiness, double vision and dizziness.

Levetiracetam

Levetiracetam is licensed for add-on treatment in partial epilepsies, but it may also be useful in other epilepsy types. The main side effects are drowsiness and dizziness, and these are dose related.

Oxcarbazepine

This drug is similar to carbamazepine. Although it has only recently been introduced in the UK, it has been available for many years in Scandinavian countries. It is effective in partial epilepsy and tonic–clonic seizures, and can worsen absences and myoclonic jerks.

Rash is an occasional side effect. Too high a dose can result in double vision, drowsiness and nausea.

Although it has similar side effects to carbamazepine, some people who cannot take carbamazepine because of side effects find oxcarbazepine acceptable.

Pregabalin
This is a novel antiepileptic drug, licensed in 2004 for add-on therapy in adults with partial epilepsy. Its main side effects are somnolence, dizziness, weight gain and unsteadiness.

Tiagabine
This antiepileptic drug is used as add-on medication in partial epilepsy. The drug's main side effects are dizziness, tremor, tiredness, depression and, occasionally, diarrhoea.

Topiramate
Topiramate can be used as add-on treatment or as monotherapy for a variety of seizure types. Its side effects usually occur on starting treatment and include tiredness, stomach upset, unsteadiness, poor concentration, word-finding difficulties and rarely kidney stones. Patients can also experience weight loss. Pins and needles are commonly experienced on starting treatment.

Vigabatrin
This drug is licensed only for partial epilepsy in combination with other antiepileptic drugs. However, it may also have some use in other forms of epilepsy in children.

About 1 in 20 people develops depression as a side effect of the drug, and occasionally confusion or psychotic symptoms can occur. Other side effects such as drowsiness and dizziness are usually mild. Some patients also put on weight while taking vigabatrin.

Long-term vigabatrin use results in varying degrees of tunnel vision in up to a third of patients. As a result of this, vigabatrin is rarely used except in cases where this risk outweighs possible benefits (for example, in some severe childhood epilepsies). People already on vigabatrin need to have their vision closely monitored by a specialist.

Zonisamide

This is the most recent drug licensed in the UK. It was licensed in 2005 as an add-on treatment for adults with partial epilepsy. The drug has, however, been available in Japan since 1989. Development in Europe and the UK was halted initially because of concerns about kidney stones.

Kidneys stones are a rare side effect. The more common side effects are stomach upset, irritability, drowsiness and dizziness. As with topiramate, weight loss can occur.

Other drugs

Drugs that have been developed primarily for other conditions (for example, diuretic drugs or drugs to treat anxiety and depression) have, in some instances, proved valuable in the treatment of epileptic seizures.

Acetazolamide

This drug is a diuretic (a drug that makes you pass more urine), and is mainly used to treat glaucoma (an eye condition). It is, however, occasionally used as additional medication for patients with epilepsy and, in some, it can be very effective.

The main problem is that after a few months tolerance develops (that is, it loses its ability to work effectively) in some patients; it can also cause a rash. The other main side effects are excessive thirst, tingling in the hands and feet, tiredness and loss of appetite.

Clobazam

This is a benzodiazepine (see 'Clonazepam' on page 62). It may be very effective in most types of epilepsy as an additional medication, but again tolerance develops in some patients after a few weeks or months.

It is occasionally given intermittently (that is, for three or four days at a time) in those whose seizures occur in small groups (clusters) or at set times (for example, at the time of menstruation), or on days when it is particularly important for the patient to avoid a seizure.

Diazepam

This drug is also a benzodiazepine and it is not usually used as regular medication, but as a one-off in order to stop a long seizure. For this purpose, it can be given by mouth or by suppository by carers or family.

Recently midazolam (another benzodiazepine), given as a solution into the nose or mouth during a seizure, has been used as an alternative. In hospital, it can be given by intravenous infusion (that is, directly into a vein) to stop prolonged seizures.

Vitamins and diets

There is little evidence that vitamins or diet can help seizures. Vitamin supplements may, however, be necessary for those on long-term antiepileptic drug treatment, because some antiepileptic drugs can interfere with the body's vitamin stores. Supplementary folic acid is also recommended for those who wish to get pregnant.

There is a high-fat, low-carbohydrate diet called a ketogenic diet that may help seizure control in some children with severe epilepsy and learning disorders. Unfortunately, this diet is unpleasant and difficult to maintain, and so is rarely used.

Drugs for the future

There are at present many studies taking place throughout the world of potential antiepileptic drugs. This is encouraging for the future of antiepileptic drug treatment. However, no drug so far has proved to be a cure all, and one of the unanswered questions for epilepsy research is why only some patients respond to only some drugs.

Nevertheless, each new drug enables a greater number of patients to show significant improvement in their epilepsy; it is hoped that, with a greater armoury of drugs, fewer people will have uncontrolled seizures.

The newer drugs may have fewer side effects than the older drugs, but it is important to realise that long-term side effects of new drugs may be unrecognised in contrast to those of older drugs, some of which have been around for over 50 years.

KEY POINTS

■ Antiepileptic medication will help control seizures in most people

■ Some of the drugs used have been around since the beginning of the twentieth century

■ Newer antiepileptic drugs may offer advantages over certain of the older therapies

Special situations

What conditions need special consideration?

There are two other types of convulsions and seizures, described below, which need to be considered. Also, pregnancy in a person with epilepsy needs careful monitoring and treatment.

Other types of convulsions and seizures

Febrile convulsions (experienced by young children) and status epilepticus seizures (a seizure that lasts more than 30 minutes) have particular characteristics that require a special explanation.

Febrile convulsions

This term is usually reserved for convulsions that occur in young children (aged three months to five years) only at the time of a fever ('febrile'). Febrile convulsions are of importance because they are common and often frightening.

A febrile convulsion should not, however, be considered to be epilepsy, because the condition

usually ceases as the child grows older and epilepsy
develops in fewer than one in ten cases.

Is there a brain infection?

It is sometimes necessary to exclude brain infections
such as meningitis as a cause. Occasionally a 'lumbar
puncture' (in which a needle is inserted into the spine
of a child in order to withdraw a sample of
cerebrospinal fluid [CSF], which is fluid that surrounds
the brain) is needed to make sure that there is no brain
infection. In most cases there is no meningitis or other
serious cause.

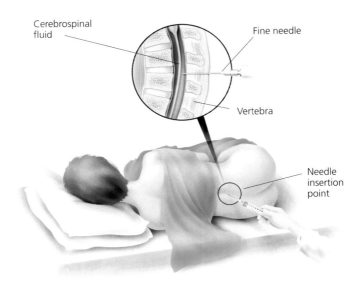

For a lumbar puncture a needle is inserted into the base of the
spine to obtain a sample of cerebrospinal fluid. Examination of
the cerebrospinal fluid can help in the diagnosis of such diseases
as meningitis.

The procedure for lumbar puncture

The patient lies on one side and a needle is inserted into the base of the spine. A small sample of CSF is withdrawn. Examination of the CSF in the laboratory can help in the diagnosis of such diseases as meningitis.

How common are febrile convulsions?

Over three per cent of children between the ages of three months and five years will have at least one seizure associated with fever without underlying brain disease. It is more common in those with a relative who has had similar seizures or who has epilepsy.

One-third of children who have a febrile convulsion have subsequent febrile convulsions, but a small number (less than five per cent) go on to develop true epilepsy.

If a child has had a convulsion with fever, then in future febrile episodes the child's temperature should be kept down with paracetamol and cold sponging. In very susceptible children diazepam suppositories can be given at the time of a fever to prevent another convulsion, and very rarely a child may need regular antiepileptic medication, usually with valproate or phenobarbital.

Keeping a child's temperature down

If a child has had a convusion with fever, the child's temperature should be kept down with paracetamol and, if necessary, a fan.

Status epilepticus

Most seizures last only a few minutes. Some, however, can persist for much longer periods – sometimes hours

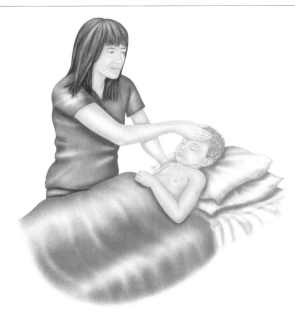

If a child has had a convulsion with fever, the child's temperature should be kept down.

or even days. This is referred to as status epilepticus, which is defined as a seizure or a series of seizures lasting more than 30 minutes in which the patient does not regain consciousness. This can apply to all seizure types.

Convulsive status epilepticus

Tonic–clonic status epilepticus (usually called convulsive status epilepticus) is of most importance because it carries a substantial risk. As many as 10 per cent of patients with convulsive status epilepticus die (usually not as a result of the epilepsy itself, but of the serious underlying cause of the status epilepticus, for example, meningitis, stroke or malignant brain tumours).

About half the patients with status epilepticus have had chronic epilepsy; in these cases sudden withdrawal of the antiepileptic drug is one of the most common identifiable causes. About half the patients have convulsive status epilepticus as their first seizure. When status epilepticus occurs, urgent hospitalisation and emergency, intravenous, antiepileptic drug therapy are required.

Many patients have increasing numbers of seizures throughout the day leading up to the convulsive status epilepticus, and in some (certainly those in whom status epilepticus occurs regularly) diazepam given by mouth or suppository will prevent its development. Such a contingency plan needs to be made between the doctor and the carers or the family of the patient.

Non-convulsive types
The other, non-convulsive types of status epilepticus are not as serious. Often the patient will just have a prolonged typical seizure or series of seizures, leading to confusion that can go on for days. Non-convulsive status epilepticus can respond well to medication given by mouth (often diazepam).

Pregnancy and epilepsy
Careful monitoring of drug levels and frequency of seizures is necessary during pregnancy to ensure the health and well-being of both mother and baby.

Conception
Women with epilepsy have lower birth rates. This is mainly as a result of social pressures, although epilepsy and its treatment can occasionally affect fertility. Furthermore, some antiepileptic drugs may have the effect of decreasing sexual drive.

The effectiveness of the contraceptive pill can be reduced by some antiepileptic drugs and higher doses of the pill may be necessary in order to provide adequate contraception (see page 49).

Pregnancy

During pregnancy, about 30 per cent of patients experience an increase in seizures, 20 per cent experience a decrease in seizures and 50 per cent experience no change. The way that the body deals with antiepileptic drugs is different during pregnancy, and regular monitoring of drug levels and seizures is often required.

Adjusting the drug dose

Sometimes the dose of antiepileptic drugs has to be changed at some point during pregnancy. It is not uncommon for the mother to decide to reduce her medication during pregnancy because of a concern about the effects of the antiepileptic drugs on the developing child. Major, convulsive seizures can, however, damage the developing child or result in miscarriage, and thus the importance of good compliance cannot be over-emphasised.

The risks of antiepileptic drugs to the development of the baby in the uterus are small but real. A balance between the effects of drugs and seizures has to be achieved, and this can be very difficult. Decisions must be tailored to individual circumstances, and the doctor should provide full information on these risks in order that the patient can make an informed choice.

Risk of abnormalities

The risk of malformations is higher in infants born to

mothers on polytherapy and on high doses of antiepileptic drugs. The overall frequency of abnormalities of the baby at birth is about one to two per cent for the general population, and four per cent for babies born to mothers on one antiepileptic drug (that is, still quite small), and up to 20 per cent for babies born to mothers on three different antiepileptic drugs (that is, quite high).

Some antiepileptic drugs may be safer than others. Recent evidence suggests that valproate is less safe than carbamazepine, and may be associated with later difficulties at school.

The most common significant abnormality in infants born to mothers with epilepsy is cleft lip/palate, which accounts for about one-third of the abnormalities seen. Spina bifida, the more serious side effect of drug treatment, is most common when the mother is taking valproate (1 to 2 per cent of births) or carbamazepine (0.5 to 1 per cent of births). Patients on these drugs can have ultrasound and blood tests during pregnancy to detect spina bifida early enough for the pregnancy to be safely terminated if the parents wish.

Vitamin supplements

It is recommended that all women should take the appropriate dose of folic acid tablets (this is a naturally occurring vitamin) before conception and throughout the first three months of pregnancy, because this reduces the risk of miscarriage and fetal malformation, especially spina bifida.

In the final stages of pregnancy vitamin K supplements should be given to the mother, and the newborn child should also receive vitamin K because antiepileptic drugs decrease the amount of this vitamin in the body. If the newborn child does not have enough vitamin K, then the blood may not clot properly, and there may be problems with bleeding and brain haemorrhage.

Breast-feeding

Women with epilepsy on antiepileptic drugs can usually breast-feed safely, because with most antiepileptic drugs very little is passed out into breast milk. The exceptions are high doses of ethosuximide or phenobarbital, which are excreted in breast milk in significant quantities; phenobarbital excreted into breast milk can make the baby drowsy.

KEY POINTS

■ Convulsions that occur in young children only at the time of a fever do not usually lead to epilepsy

■ Seizures that last for hours or days are known as status epilepticus, and convulsive status epilepticus is a medical emergency

■ During pregnancy the risks of antiepileptic drugs to the baby are small, and smaller than the risks of having uncontrolled convulsions

■ It is generally safe for women to breast-feed while taking antiepileptic drugs

Social implications

What effect does epilepsy have on daily life?

Although we have spent a large part of this book dealing with the medical aspects of epilepsy, it is important to realise that there are many social implications of epilepsy, for instance with regard to:

- driving

- schooling

- employment

- relationships.

Unfortunately, society still places extra pressures on those who have epilepsy, sometimes with some justification as in the case of driving.

Driving

Seizures while driving are still one of the most common preventable causes of road traffic accidents. The rules laid down about driving are straightforward.

Informing the DVLA

It is the obligation and responsibility of every person who has any condition that may impede his or her driving (this includes all people with epilepsy) to inform the Driver and Vehicle Licensing Agency (DVLA).

Anyone who fails to inform the DVLA, and continues to drive, is committing an offence. Furthermore, failing to inform the DVLA may invalidate the driving insurance. This applies to all people with seizures, and for this purpose even the smallest epileptic event (for example, an aura or a myoclonic jerk) is counted as a seizure.

Reapplying for a licence

Once the DVLA has been informed, the patient should stop driving and can reapply for a licence only when one of the criteria in the box on page 83 has been fulfilled.

After a single epileptic seizure or if there is loss of consciousness of no known cause, patients can also be barred from driving for one year. When reapplying for a licence, it is necessary for the patient to fill in a detailed form about the attacks, and the DVLA can also seek information from the patient's GP and hospital specialist. If any person is unhappy with the DVLA's decision, it is possible to appeal through a Magistrates' court.

Coming off medication

If a patient has been seizure free and has thus regained his or her driving licence, but wishes to come off medication, it is advised that the patient should not drive during the changes in medication and for six months after the withdrawal, although this is not

DVLA criteria for driving

The DVLA should be told of any condition that may impede driving. You will then have to reapply for an ordinary driving licence but must fulfil one of the criteria:

- No epileptic attacks (this also includes aura) have occurred during the previous year

- Epileptic attacks have occurred in the last three years only during periods of sleep

legally binding. Unfortunately, a seizure that occurs while coming off medication will result in loss of the licence.

Other types of licence

The rules for large goods vehicle (LGV) and passenger-carrying vehicle (PCV) licences are much stricter, and it is not possible to hold these licences if a person has a continuing liability to epileptic seizures.

This is interpreted for the HGV licence as meaning no epileptic seizure or antiepileptic medication for the previous ten years and no medical evidence of a continuing risk of seizures (for example, three per second spike and wave on the EEG or a brain abnormality on a brain scan).

Employment
Jobs barred to people with epilepsy

There are a few occupations that are barred by statutory provision for people with epilepsy, and these are:

- aircraft pilot

- ambulance driver

- taxi driver

- train driver

- merchant seaman

- armed services.

Risks and discrimination

There are also certain jobs that involve substantial risks if a seizure should occur and thus cannot be recommended (for example, scaffolder), and common sense should apply when considering such jobs. Overall, however, epilepsy is covered by the Disability Discrimination Act 2005, which means that people with epilepsy should not be discriminated against when applying for any job.

When to tell people at work

Patients are under an obligation to tell employers if they have epilepsy, if this could affect their ability to do the job or affect their safety at work. Failure to disclose epilepsy in such circumstances can be used as grounds for dismissal.

If a seizure is likely to occur at work, it is, in the authors' view, usually better to tell an employer rather than keep the epilepsy secret. If an employer is aware of a person's epilepsy and takes it into consideration, then the work insurance will cover that person regardless of his or her condition. It is important to tell a workmate if a seizure is likely to occur at work, and to explain what to do if a seizure should occur.

Applying for a job

When initially applying for a job, unless the epilepsy is likely to have a severe effect on the ability to do the job, there is no obligation to inform possible employers unless specifically asked. If asked on forms, it is important not to over-emphasise the epilepsy and in some cases it may be advisable to leave that section blank or to write that it will be discussed at interview.

The best moments for mentioning epilepsy are just before accepting the job offer or at final interview, but again it is important to try to place it in a favourable light. Often a letter from the GP or hospital doctor helps.

The prejudice perceived by people with epilepsy when applying for jobs is sometimes greater than the actual prejudice. Some people blame their failure to get work on their epilepsy when, in fact, the problem lies more in the person's attitude – it is essential at interview to appear confident, and appropriate for the job, rather than dwell too much on the negative aspects of epilepsy.

Assessing the risks

One of the most important features of epilepsy is that it is an intermittent condition. If someone has a seizure once a week (this would be considered as poorly controlled epilepsy), it still leaves 313 days in a year when the person is seizure free.

It is thus important that a person does not let the epilepsy take over and dictate his or her life. Over-protection, excessive restrictions and under-achievement are far too common secondary handicaps of epilepsy, which can be avoided.

Leisure activities

The main dangers from epilepsy come from its unpredictability, and certain precautions need to be taken. It would be prudent to avoid certain high-risk situations such as mountain climbing, scuba diving and hang gliding (although well-organised mountain climbs are possible).

In most other circumstances the social and psychological damage done by restricting a person's life probably outstrips the risks. Swimming is perfectly possible, but preferably with someone who knows about the epilepsy and knows what to do should a seizure occur, and the pool attendant should be informed.

Cycling and horse riding are perfectly possible, but again attention should be paid to the possible risks. Both should be pursued either with someone who knows about the epilepsy or in an organised group, and a helmet is mandatory.

Leisure activities and epilepsy

Many activities may be undertaken and should be encouraged. The main dangers from epilepsy come from its unpredictability and so precautions need to be taken.

Safety at home

At home, most activities carry only a small risk. There are, however, certain actions that can be taken to minimise these risks. Showers should be preferred to baths and, if a bath is taken, it should be shallow and someone should be informed. In addition, the bathroom door should remain unlocked.

A microwave is preferable to a cooker, and pans of hot oil should be avoided. Guards for open fires,

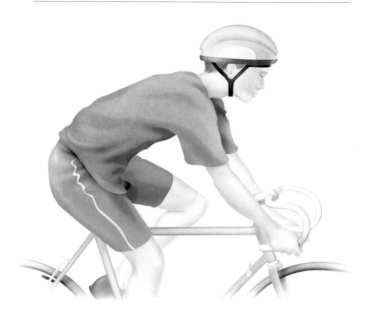

The main dangers from epilepsy come from its unpredictability and precautions need to be taken.

radiators and cookers are advisable. Last, there are alarms that are available for people with epilepsy, which are triggered if, for example, the person falls; these are useful for people with frequent seizures who are living alone.

Danger of frequent falls

Frequent falls in someone with poorly controlled epilepsy can cause head and facial injuries. If these falls are repeated often, then a certain amount of brain damage and facial scarring can occur. In these people (very much the minority of people who have epilepsy), a protective helmet is advisable.

Schooling and parenting

It is wrong to generalise about a child with epilepsy. Epilepsy, as we hope is now apparent, describes many different conditions, has many different underlying causes and occurs in many different people.

It is inexcusable to label a person with epilepsy as an epileptic child or an epileptic adult, and thus to suggest a stereotype. Despite this, there are some important points about schooling that need to be made.

Most children with epilepsy attend normal schools, and only the minority, who have epilepsy and learning difficulties or very severe epilepsy, need to attend special schools (advice about these is available from a number of organisations – see 'Useful addresses' on pages 103–13). Despite attending mainstream education many children with epilepsy under-achieve at school for a variety of reasons.

Ability to learn and concentrate

Epilepsy itself and antiepileptic drugs can impair a child's ability to learn. However, with modern drug management, there is less impairment of memory and greater control of seizures.

A child with absence epilepsy can have many seizures that are unrecognised by both child and teacher, but which can present as lapses of concentration and poor class performance. Seizures at night can also affect performance during the day.

Low expectations

More importantly, many children with epilepsy are almost expected by some to perform poorly, and this expectation by parents and teachers soon becomes self-fulfilling. Poor school attendance, low self-esteem and anxieties about school are all likely to be major factors.

There has to be good communication among school, parents, child and doctor. It is important that the school knows about the epilepsy, and that teachers know what to do about seizures and understand a child's condition. Education packages for schools are available from a number of charitable organisations (see 'Useful addresses', pages 103–13).

Over-protection

In addition, it is important that neither teachers nor parents restrict the activities of a child unnecessarily (see 'Assessing the risks', page 85). The child should be encouraged to think positively and to take part in school activities. Teachers should be aware of possible teasing and bullying.

If it is likely that a child will have a seizure at school, then often it is worth educating the class about seizures and epilepsy. It is important that the child does not feel, or indeed become, isolated because of his or her seizures.

Over-protection by families, even in well-controlled epilepsy, let alone in poorly controlled epilepsy, is very common and is counterproductive. This over-protection, which often persists into adulthood, can result in social isolation, poor social graces, dependency, childishness, under-achievement and low self-esteem.

Striking a balance is understandably difficult, but it is important that this issue is not ignored. Parents should not be afraid to discuss their child's epilepsy with doctors, counsellors or others in order to have a better understanding not only of their child's epilepsy, but also of the restrictions that this will impose on their child's life.

In our experience, parents tend to verge much too much on the side of over-vigilance and over-anxiety, and thus the potential for psychological and social damage is great.

Relationships

In broad terms, people with epilepsy have fewer relationships and are often more isolated than is normal. Prejudice among the general public is often blamed, but, although prejudice is undoubtedly a factor, the causes may be more complex.

What gets in the way?

Cultural aspects are important and factors such as low self-esteem and fear of prejudice may result in a perception of greater prejudice than is actually present. This can lead to anxiety over forming relationships and consequential social isolation and a vicious circle result. We often find that these worries remain even when patients become seizure free.

Positive thinking

Taking control of one's life is important. Many people with epilepsy need to be encouraged to think positively about themselves and their condition, and to face their anxieties. Occasionally help is needed, and advice about this is available from a number of sources (see 'Useful addresses' on pages 103–13). It is important not to let epilepsy dominate one's life inappropriately, as such a preoccupation can be very self-destructive.

Telling your partner

Once in a relationship, if the epilepsy is still active, it is important that the partner is aware of this. There is no evidence to suggest that knowledge of a person's epilepsy is a major cause in the break-up of relationships. Although this may sound an obvious recommendation, we are certainly aware of one person whose wife discovered about his epilepsy for the first time during a honeymoon night.

How and when to tell a partner can be difficult, but again the positive aspects of the condition should be emphasised – usually epilepsy is easily controlled, it is not inherited, it does not lead to mental illness, etc. It is also perfectly possible to have a family (see 'Pregnancy and epilepsy', pages 76–8), and for people with active epilepsy to look after and bring up children.

There is a danger of over-dependency in some relationships, and of treating the affected partner as a child. Both of these should be avoided.

Psychiatric disease
Is epilepsy a form of psychiatric disease?
The connection between psychiatric disease and seizures is complex. In the past, epilepsy was viewed as a form of psychiatric disease, but now it is considered a physical brain disease.

Is psychiatric disease common in epilepsy?
Psychiatric disease is, however, not uncommon in people with epilepsy. A person with epilepsy faces many social pressures, and is more likely to be unemployed and single. It is thus not surprising that anxiety and depression are common in those with epilepsy, especially those with a long history of poorly controlled seizures.

Both seizures and antiepileptic drugs can, however, compound this depression through their effects on the brain, and can occasionally produce a very severe depression that may require hospitalisation and drug treatment.

Rarely, patients with temporal lobe epilepsy have episodes of paranoia and schizophrenic-like illnesses. These episodes are usually short-lived, occurring around the time of a seizure, just after a seizure or between seizures. In a few individuals, these episodes may persist and may require long-term drug treatment.

The exact association between temporal lobe epilepsy and psychosis is complex, and both increases in seizure frequency (flurries of seizures) and decreases in seizure frequency can in some cases result in psychotic episodes in some unfortunate people.

Some psychiatric diseases and epilepsy have a common cause, for instance severe brain damage at birth may lead to seizures, personality problems and psychiatric disease. In these cases, it is not the epilepsy that causes the psychiatric problems but the underlying cause that results in both.

KEY POINTS

■ All people who have a driving licence need to inform the DVLA if they develop epileptic seizures

■ It is advisable to inform an employer if you have epilepsy

■ High-risk situations such as strenuous or dangerous sports should be avoided; most sports can be enjoyed under some supervision

■ Parents of children with epilepsy should not be over-protective because this can result in social isolation

■ Forming relationships can occasionally be difficult for people with epilepsy, but they must be careful not to let the condition 'control' their lives

Overall outlook

How will epilepsy affect life?

With the appropriate care and treatment, most people with epilepsy can look forward to leading a normal and fulfilling life, with a normal life expectancy.

What is the likely outcome?

As was described in the introduction, epilepsy resolves in most people, and can thus be said to have a good outlook (prognosis). About 80 per cent of people on antiepileptic medication become seizure free, and there thus has to be the decision about when to stop the medication.

It is usual to wait for a patient to be seizure free for roughly two years before stopping medication. There are a number of factors that determine the chances of success or failure in withdrawing drugs, including the underlying cause of the epilepsy, the type of epilepsy, the length of the history and the EEG findings. Overall, however, about 60 per cent of patients who have been seizure free for two years successfully come off drugs.

The chances of coming off medication are better in young people, and in those taking only one antiepileptic drug. Some people do not wish to risk coming off their drugs, because the social consequences of having a seizure may be too great (loss of driving licence, etc.).

These social consequences tend to be greater in adults than in children. Indeed, because of the better chances of withdrawing medication, the lesser consequences of having a seizure and the effects of medication on schooling, seizure-free children are often the group that benefit most from attempting to discontinue their antiepileptic drug therapy.

Mental and physical health

There is often concern that epilepsy and seizures will lead to mental and physical deterioration. This does not usually happen. In most cases, seizures either stop or are well controlled by antiepileptic drugs, and these people can lead normal lives.

Unfortunately, there are a few who have uncontrolled seizures, in whom changes do occur. In these cases, however, the deterioration is usually the result of the underlying cause of the epilepsy or injuries that occur during the seizures rather than the seizures themselves.

The development of mental illness is often another concern, but, as has already been explained, mental illness directly attributable to seizures is rare, and seizures themselves rarely lead to the destruction of personality or mind.

Death and epilepsy

In poorly controlled, severe epilepsy, there is a small

but definite risk of injury or death. The reasons for this are complex. In patients whose epilepsy is caused by a serious brain disorder, for instance stroke or tumour, life expectancy can be shortened by the underlying condition.

People with epilepsy are at a higher risk of accidents usually while having a seizure or as the result of the seizure. There may also be socioeconomic factors at play.

Sudden unexpected death in a previously healthy person for which no cause is found *post mortem* is more common in epilepsy (approximately 1 in 500 people with epilepsy per year) than in the general population. The deaths usually occur in the wake of unwitnessed convulsive seizures and may be the result of impaired breathing after the attack. It is important to emphasise that this is a rare eventuality (there is approximately 1 death per 5,000 convulsive seizures).

It is certain, however, that people with well-controlled epilepsy do better than those with poorly controlled epilepsy and, as our treatment of epilepsy continues to improve, so the prognosis for epilepsy, the lives of those with epilepsy and even the life expectancy of those with epilepsy improve along with it.

KEY POINTS

- Epilepsy resolves in most people

- People with epilepsy can control or stop their seizures with drugs and can then lead normal lives

- Most seizures are entirely innocent, rarely causing brain damage or death

Finally

In this book there are a number of important points that we would like to emphasise:

- Epilepsy is a common and treatable condition.

- A seizure results from an 'electrical storm' in the brain, and the form of a seizure depends on where it starts and how far it spreads.

- A number of conditions can be confused with seizures.

- There are a multitude of causes of seizures.

- Febrile convulsions rarely lead to epilepsy.

- Most people with epilepsy are well controlled with drug treatment, which must be taken regularly.

- Doses of antiepileptic drugs are determined by the balance of seizure control against drug side effects.

- Antiepileptic blood levels are merely a guide to drug doses.

- Epilepsy gets better and 'goes away' in many people.

- The prognosis probably relates mainly to the underlying cause of the epilepsy.

- Brain surgery is successful in, and suitable for, a number of patients with drug-resistant epilepsy.

- Most prejudice against people with epilepsy is unjust, but often it is not as great as the person with epilepsy believes.

- Most people with epilepsy should lead normal lives, and should not be over-protected.

- Last, epileptic is an adjective that should be confined to the phrase 'epileptic seizure' and not be used to describe and stereotype people.

Glossary

amytal test: one of the tests carried out before epilepsy surgery. It consists of the injection of sodium amytal (an anaesthetic) into the blood supply in each half of the brain in turn to determine the possible effects of epilepsy surgery on memory and language

aura: the warning that may occur before a major seizure or in isolation; it is a simple partial seizure

compliance: the act of taking a drug as instructed

computed tomography (CT): a scan using X-rays and computer analysis to form pictures of slices through the organ being scanned

dysplasia: congenital abnormalities caused by abnormal development of the brain

electroencephalography: the recording of brain waves (the electrical activity within the brain); an EEG is an electroencephalogram or -graph

epileptic seizures: also known as fits and can be

thought of as an electrical storm in the brain. They are categorised into partial seizures (simple partial, complex partial and secondary generalised), which begin in one part of the brain but can spread to other parts, and generalised seizures (tonic–clonic, clonic, tonic, absences and myoclonus), which begin in both halves of the brain at once

febrile convulsions: fits that occur in children at the time of fever; they rarely lead to epilepsy

hemispheres of the brain: the two halves of the brain, in most of us the left hemisphere is 'dominant' and controls language

hippocampus: a part of the temporal lobe (see 'lobes of the brain'), which is involved in the formation of memories and which if damaged commonly causes epilepsy

hyperventilation: over-breathing, which can occasionally be confused with an epileptic seizure

idiosyncratic side effects: allergic side effects – the most common being a rash

lobes of the brain: anatomical divisions of the brain. Each lobe has a particular set of functions: the frontal lobe is at the front and deals with movement, the parietal lobe is in the middle and deals with sensation, the occipital lobe is at the back and deals with sight, and the temporal lobe is at the side and deals with memory formation

magnetic resonance imaging (MRI): a form of scanning that relies on a strong magnetic field and radio waves. It provides a very detailed picture of the brain. MRI is much better than CT at detecting brain abnormalities that cause epilepsy

monotherapy: the taking of one drug

pharmacoresistant epilepsy: also known as refractory or drug-resistant epilepsy and is epilepsy that does not respond to antiepileptic drug therapy

photosensitivity: present in about 1 in 20 people with epilepsy. It is the propensity to have a seizure brought on by flashing lights

polytherapy: the taking of two or more drugs

prognosis: a term used to refer to the outcome of a condition.

pseudo-seizures: seizures that are not epileptic but which have an emotional or psychological basis. They do not respond to antiepileptic drug treatment, and can be difficult to tell apart from epileptic seizures

status epilepticus: a seizure, or series of seizures, without consciousness being regained that continues for over 30 minutes. If the seizure is a convulsion (convulsive status epilepticus), there is a significant risk of injury, and this should be treated as an emergency

syncope: a faint

video telemetry: the simultaneous recording of an EEG with video; used in attacks that are difficult to diagnose and for assessment before epilepsy surgery

Useful addresses

Where can I find out more?

We have included the following organisations because, on preliminary investigation, they may be of use to the reader. However, we do not have first-hand experience of each organisation and so cannot guarantee the organisation's integrity. The reader must therefore exercise his or her own discretion and judgement when making further enquiries.

Benefits Enquiry Line

Tel: 0800 882200
Minicom: 0800 243355
Website: www.dwp.gov.uk
N Ireland: 0800 220674
NI minicom: 0800 243789

Government agency giving information and advice on sickness and disability benefits for people with disabilities and their carers.

Brainwave – The Irish Epilepsy Association
249 Crumlin Road
Dublin 12, Eire
Tel: 00 353 1455 7500
Fax: 00 353 1455 7013
Helpline: 00 353 1455 4133 (9.30am–1pm Wed only)
Email: info@epilepsy.ie
Website: www.epilepsy.ie

Provides help, information and support for everyone
with epilepsy, their families and carers. Literature, self-
help groups and specialist nurses also available.

Citizens Advice Bureaux
Myddelton House, 115–123 Pentonville Road
London N1 9LZ
Tel: 020 7833 2181 (admin only)
Website: www.adviceguide.org.uk

HQ of national charity offering a wide variety of
practical, financial and legal advice. Network of local
charities throughout the UK listed in phone books and
in *Yellow Pages* under 'C'.

Croydon Epilepsy Society
Len Pyant Community Centre, 17 Elmwood Road
Croydon CR0 2SN
Tel: 020 8665 1255 (Tues–Fri 10am–3pm)

Day centre for people with epilepsy and learning
difficulties. Offers advice and information on all aspects
of epilepsy and helps with form filling, benefits claims
and advocacy when dealing with other agencies.

David Lewis Centre

Mill Lane, Warford
Nr Alderley Edge, Cheshire SK9 7UD
Tel: 01565 640000
Fax: 01565 640100
Email: enquiries@davidlewis.org.uk
Website: www.davidlewis.org.uk

Provides assessment, respite and long-term care and education for children and adults with severe epilepsy and learning difficulties. Rehabilitation unit offers service to children suffering accidental brain injury. Referral necessary.

Driver and Vehicle Licensing Agency (DVLA)

Driver Medical Section
Swansea SA6 7JL
Helpline: 0870 600 0301 (8am–5.30pm)
Website: dvla.gov.uk

Government office offering advice to drivers with medical conditions.

Enlighten – Action for Epilepsy

5 Coates Place
Edinburgh EH3 7AA
Tel: 0131 226 5458
Fax: 0131 220 2855
Email: info@enlighten.org.uk
Website: www.enlighten.org.uk

Centre providing information, training and advocacy for anyone directly or indirectly affected by epilepsy. Offers holistic help through support groups and befriending service.

Epilepsy Action

New Anstey House, Gate Way Drive
Yeadon, Leeds LS19 7XY
Tel: 0113 210 8800
Fax: 0113 391 0300
Helpline: 0808 800 5050
Email: epilepsy@epilepsy.org.uk
Website: www.epilepsy.org.uk

Provides help, information and advice for everyone with epilepsy, their families and carers. Literature, self-help groups throughout the UK and specialist nurses also available.

Epilepsy Bereaved

PO Box 112, Wantage, Oxfordshire OX12 8XT
Tel: 01235 772850
Fax: 01235 772850
Helpline: 01235 772852
Email: epilepsybereaved@dial.pipex.com
Website: www.sudep.org

Working towards prevention of deaths from epilepsy, including sudden unexpected death in epilepsy (SUDEP), by raising awareness and promoting research. Provides information and support to people bereaved by epilepsy.

Epilepsy Connections

100 Wellington Street
Glasgow G2 6DH
Tel: 0141 248 4125
Fax: 0141 248 5887
Email: info@epilepsyconnections.org.uk
Website: www.epilepsyconnections.org.uk

Offers a range of information and support to families affected by epilepsy through training and field workers in the community with various short-term projects.

Epilepsy Research Foundation
PO Box 3004
London W4 4XT
Tel: 020 8995 4781
Fax: 020 8995 4781
Email: info@erf.org.uk
Website: www.erf.org.uk

Funds research into the causes, treatment and prevention of epilepsy.

Epilepsy Scotland
48 Govan Road, Glasgow G51 1JL
Tel: 0141 427 4911
Fax: 0141 419 1709
Helpline: 0808 800 2200 (Mon–Fri 10am–4pm, Thurs 10am–6pm)
Email: enquiries@epilepsyscotland.org.uk
Website: www.epilepsyscotland.org.uk

Provides advice, information, training services, literature and has support groups.

Epilepsy Wales
PO Box 4168
Cardiff CF14 0WZ
Tel: 029 2075 5515
Helpline: 0845 741 3774
Email: epilepsywales@aol.com
Website: epilepsy-wales.co.uk

Provides advice, information and training with field workers. Has local self-help groups.

FABLE (For a Better Life With Epilepsy)
Lower Ground Floor, 305 Glossop Road
Sheffield S10 2HL
Tel: 0114 275 5335
Fax: 0114 275 6444
Helpline: 0800 521629
Email: fable@btconnect.com
Website: www.fable.org.uk

Funds vagus nerve stimulation therapy. Offers help and support via patient database to put people in touch with each other.

Fund for Epilepsy
38 Buckingham Palace Road
London SW1W 0RE
Tel: 020 7592 3270
Fax: 020 7821 5000
Email: ffe@epilepsyfund.org.uk
Website: www.epilepsyfund.org.uk

Raises funds for research into the causes and cure for epilepsy.

Joint Epilepsy Council
PO Box 186
Leeds LS20 8WY
Tel: 01943 871852
Fax: 01943 873592
Email: sharon.jec@btconnect.com
Website: www.jointepilepsycouncil.org.uk

Umbrella membership organisation for the voluntary sector listing local services available around the UK on its website. Presents evidence-based views on the need to improve standards in health and social care and education.

Mersey Region Epilepsy Association

Neurosupport Centre, Norton Street
Liverpool L3 8LR
Tel: 0151 298 2666
Fax: 0151 298 2333
Email: epilepsy@mrea.demon.co.uk
Website: www.epilepsymersey.org.uk

Provides advice, information, literature, lectures, counselling and has network of self-help groups in Merseyside and Cheshire.

NHS Direct

Tel: 0845 4647 (24 hours a day, 365 days a year)
Textphone: 0845 606 4647
Website: www.nhsdirect.nhs.uk
NHS Scotland: 0800 224488

Offers confidential health-care advice, information and referral service. A good first port of call for any health advice.

NHS Smoking Helpline

Tel: 0800 169 0169 (7am–11pm, 365 days a year)
Website: www.givingupsmoking.co.uk
Pregnancy smoking helpline: 0800 169 9169
(12noon–9pm, 365 days a year)

Scotland: 0800 848484
(12noon–12midnight, 365 days a year)
N. Ireland: 0800 858585
(12noon–11pm, 365 days a year)
Wales: 0800 085 2219

Have advice, help and encouragement on giving up
smoking. Specialist advisers available to offer on-going
support to those who genuinely are trying to give up
smoking. Can refer to local branches.

National Centre for Young People with Epilepsy

St Piers School and College, St Piers Lane
Lingfield, Surrey RH7 6PW
Tel: 01342 832243
Fax: 01342 834639
Email: info@ncype.org.uk
Website: www.ncype.org.uk

Residential school for young adults and children with
severe epilepsy. Medical centre provides assessment
with psychological, physiotherapy, occupational and
speech therapies. Referral for people using the NHS in
England and Wales.

National Institute for Health and Clinical Excellence (NICE)

MidCity Place, 71 High Holborn
London WC1V 6NA
Tel: 020 7067 5800
Fax: 020 7067 5801
Email: nice@nice.org.uk
Website: www.nice.org.uk

Provides national guidance on the promotion of good health and the prevention and treatment of ill-health. Patient information leaflets are available for each piece of guidance issued.

National Society for Epilepsy
Chesham Lane
Chalfont St Peter, Bucks SL9 0RJ
Tel: 01494 601300
Fax: 01494 871927
Helpline: 01494 601400 (Mon-Fri 10am–4pm)
Email: information@epilepsynse.org.uk
Website: www.epilepsynse.org.uk

Provides assessment, respite and residential care for adults with severe epilepsy. Does research, provides training courses for employers, schools and others who work or live with people with epilepsy. Offers publications and videos.

Park Hospital for Children
Old Road, Headington
Oxford OX3 7LQ
Tel: 01865 741717
Fax: 01865 226355

NHS hospital providing assessment for children with severe epilepsy, often with associated learning difficulties. Referral required.

Prodigy Website
Sowerby Centre for Health Informatics at Newcastle (SCHIN), Bede House, All Saints Business Centre
Newcastle upon Tyne NE1 2ES

Tel: 0191 243 6100
Fax: 0191 243 6101
Email: prodigy-enquiries@schin.co.uk
Website: www.prodigy.nhs.uk

A website mainly for GPs giving information for patients listed by disease plus named self-help organisations.

Quit (Smoking Quitlines)
211 Old Street
London EC1V 9NR
Helpline: 0800 002200 (9am–9pm, 365 days a year)
Tel: 020 7251 1551
Fax: 020 7251 1661
Email: info@quit.org.uk
Website: www.quit.org.uk

Offers individual advice on giving up smoking in English and Asian languages. Talks to schools on smoking and can refer to local support groups. Runs training courses for professionals.

St Elizabeth's Centre
South End
Much Hadham, Herts SG10 6EW
Tel: 01279 843451
Fax: 01279 842918
Email: enquiries@stelizabeths.org.uk
Website: www.stelizabeths.org.uk

School, day college and residential home for people with epilepsy. School caters for young people between 5 and 19 years. College caters for 19–25 year olds.

Residential home offers respite and long-term care for adults. Satellite centres being developed. Referral necessary.

Westhaven – Church of Scotland
2 Upper Bourtree Drive, High Burn South
Glasgow G73 4EH
Tel: 0141 634 4563
Fax: 0141 634 0599
Email: westhaven.cos@uk.uumail.com

Assessment and rehabilitation unit for adults with epilepsy. Offers support within the community for people of all denominations. Referral needed.

The internet as a further source of information

After reading this book, you may feel that you would like further information on the subject. The internet is of course an excellent place to look and there are many websites with useful information about medical disorders, related charities and support groups.

For those who do not have a computer at home some bars and cafes offer facilities for accessing the internet. These are listed in the *Yellow Pages* under 'Internet Bars and Cafes' and 'Internet Providers'. Your local library offers a similar facility and has staff to help you find the information that you need.

It should always be remembered, however, that the internet is unregulated and anyone is free to set up a website and add information to it. Many websites offer impartial advice and information that has been compiled and checked by qualified medical professionals. Some, on the other hand, are run by commercial organisations with the purpose of promoting their own products. Others still are run by pressure groups, some of which will provide carefully assessed and accurate information whereas others may be suggesting medications or treatments that are not supported by the medical and scientific community.

Unless you know the address of the website you want to visit – for example, www.familydoctor.co.uk – you may find the following guidelines useful when searching the internet for information.

Search engines and other searchable sites

Google (www.google.co.uk) is the most popular search engine used in the UK, followed by Yahoo! (http://uk.yahoo.com) and MSN (www.msn.co.uk). Also popular are the search engines provided by Internet Service Providers such as Tiscali and other sites such as the BBC site (www.bbc.co.uk).

In addition to the search engines that index the whole web, there are also medical sites with search facilities, which act almost like mini-search engines, but cover only medical topics or even a particular area of medicine. Again, it is wise to look at who is responsible for compiling the information offered to ensure that it is impartial and medically accurate. The NHS Direct site (www.nhsdirect. nhs.uk) is an example of a searchable medical site.

Links to many British medical charities can be found at the Association of Medical Research Charities' website (www.amrc.org.uk) and at Charity Choice (www.charitychoice.co.uk).

Search phrases

Be specific when entering a search phrase. Searching for information on 'cancer' will return results for many different types of cancer as well as on cancer in general. You may even find sites offering astrological information. More useful results will be returned by using search phrases such as 'lung cancer' and 'treatments for lung cancer'. Both Google and Yahoo! offer an advanced search option that includes the ability to search for the exact phrase, enclosing the search phrase in quotes, that is, 'treatments for lung cancer' will have the same effect. Limiting a search to an exact phrase reduces the number of results returned but it is best to refine a search to an exact match only if you are not getting useful results with a normal search. Adding 'UK' to your search term will bring up mainly British sites, so a good phrase might be 'lung cancer' UK (don't include UK within the quotes). Always remember the internet is international and unregulated. It holds a wealth of valuable information but individual sites may be biased, out of date or just plain wrong. Family Doctor Publications accepts no responsibility for the content of links published in this series.

Index

Your pages

We have included the following pages because they may help you manage your illness or condition and its treatment.

Before an appointment with a health professional, it can be useful to write down a short list of questions of things that you do not understand, so that you can make sure that you do not forget anything.

Some of the sections may not be relevant to your circumstances.

We are always pleased to receive constructive criticism or suggestions about how to improve the books. You can contact us at:

Email: familydoctor@btinternet.com
Letter: Family Doctor Publications
         PO Box 4664
         Poole
         BH15 1NN

Thank you

Health-care contact details

Name:

Job title:

Place of work:

Tel:

Name:

Job title:

Place of work:

Tel:

Name:

Job title:

Place of work:

Tel:

Name:

Job title:

Place of work:

Tel:

Significant past health events – illnesses/ operations/investigations/treatments

Event	Month	Year	Age (at time)

Appointments for health care

Name:

Place:

Date:

Time:

Tel:

Name:

Place:

Date:

Time:

Tel:

Name:

Place:

Date:

Time:

Tel:

Name:

Place:

Date:

Time:

Tel:

Appointments for health care

Name:

Place:

Date:

Time:

Tel:

Name:

Place:

Date:

Time:

Tel:

Name:

Place:

Date:

Time:

Tel:

Name:

Place:

Date:

Time:

Tel:

Current medication(s) prescribed by your doctor

Medicine name:

Purpose:

Frequency & dose:

Start date:

End date:

Medicine name:

Purpose:

Frequency & dose:

Start date:

End date:

Medicine name:

Purpose:

Frequency & dose:

Start date:

End date:

Medicine name:

Purpose:

Frequency & dose:

Start date:

End date:

Other medicines/supplements you are taking, not prescribed by your doctor

Medicine/treatment:

Purpose:

Frequency & dose:

Start date:

End date:

Medicine/treatment:

Purpose:

Frequency & dose:

Start date:

End date:

Medicine/treatment:

Purpose:

Frequency & dose:

Start date:

End date:

Medicine/treatment:

Purpose:

Frequency & dose:

Start date:

End date:

Questions to ask at appointments
(Note: do bear in mind that doctors work under great time
pressure, so long lists may not be helpful for either of you)

Questions to ask at appointments
(Note: do bear in mind that doctors work under great time
pressure, so long lists may not be helpful for either of you)

Notes

Notes

Notes